MW00683076

"Want to enjoy chocolate without guilt or blowing your caloric allowance? This book is for you! A terrific blend of entertainment and information, the book reviews sound nutrition principles while teaching the reader how to enjoy the ultimate eating satisfaction of CHOCOLATE! Definitely one for the chocolate lovers!"

— Olivia Bennett Wood, M.P.H., R.D., CD Associate Professor of Dietetics, Department of Foods and Nutrition, Purdue University, and winner of the Award for Excellence in the Practice of Dietetic Education, The American Dietetic Association, October 2000

"With a wonderful sense of humor, Dr. John Ashton and Suzy Ashton take us on a guided tour into 'chocolate heaven,' unraveling the health benefits of high-quality chocolate. The authors possess a unique skill in turning scientific facts into practical, useful knowledge, making this book a must for chocolate lovers."

— Susanne Kölare, D.D.S., Ph.D., Faculty of Medicine, Karolinska Institute, Stockholm

"Everything in moderation and that ought to include chocolate. Suzy and John Ashton have explained clearly and simply the scientific reasons why chocolate is good for health. They leave no stone unturned, discussing every aspect from acne to trans-fatty acids."

— Jennie Brand-Miller, Ph.D., Professor in Human Nutrition, University of Sydney, and senior author of the international bestselling book on carbohydrates, *The G.I. Factor*

A CHOCOLATE a Day
Keeps the Doctor Away

A **CHOCOLATE** a Day
Keeps the Doctor Away

Dr. John Ashton and Suzy Ashton

Thomas Dunne Books
St. Martin's Press

New York

THOMAS DUNNE BOOKS.
An imprint of St. Martin's Press.

www.stmartins.com

Book design by Nick Wunder

ISBN 0-312-30757-8

First published in Australia by Thorsons, an imprint of HarperCollins
Publishers

First U.S. Edition: February 2003

10 9 8 7 6 5 4 3 2 1

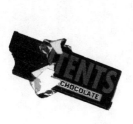

A **CHOCOLATE** a Day
Keeps the Doctor Away

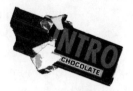

Introduction

A shiny wrapper sparkles at you as you browse through the supermarket shelves. The glittering foil catches your eye but you steel yourself against it. You remember past experiences of that smooth, sweet taste melting on your tongue. Suddenly you are jerked back to reality and you desperately think: "No! I can't give in! I can't eat . . . that!"

Have you ever experienced this feeling? As you pick up this book, are you thinking: "How can it be possible that chocolate is good for you?" Surely the authors can't be serious. Have you learned somewhere that chocolate makes you fat?

And what about the caffeine? We've all heard stories like this and at many times I'm sure we've all felt guilty when we've given in and enjoyed selecting from that box of chocolates. Feeling the chocolate melt on the palate of our mouths and savoring many of the delicious, subtle, fine flavors that chocolate has to offer, is a delightful experience. This experience, however, is often bittersweet. You've enjoyed the moment, looked back and said, "I shouldn't have done that." Guilt kicks in and you look remorsefully at the remaining (if there are any!) chocolates in the box.

In a popular women's magazine there was an article titled "Help! I need my chockie-o'clock fix!" The doctor quoted in this article said that women would feel better if they ignored their chockie cravings and went for a short walk instead. While we are not underestimating the health benefits of fresh air and exercise, the health benefits of chocolate should not be overlooked, either. Women's magazines are full of articles on weight loss and body image. In most of these chocolate is shown as a "baddie" in the fight against weight gain. This unfortunately adds to our angst when we feel the urge to splurge on chocolate.

The Appeal of Chocolate

What is it about chocolate that makes it so appealing? Roald Dahl didn't choose to call his famous children's book "Charlie and the Cabbage Factory"; and most people aren't weaned off strawberry milk before they start drinking the more adult beverage of coffee. In fact, a chocolate beverage of some sort has been offered directly beneath coffee on the menu in just about every café I've been to. And what about you? When was the last time you partook of this delightfully indulgent food? And how did you feel? Great . . . or guilty? With so much emphasis being placed on health it's no wonder that we're being encouraged to seek "healthier" snack foods than chocolate. I tried this out one day after a particularly bad day at work. Looking through the fridge I spied a bunch of celery . . . its brilliant green stems just begging to be eaten. To the side of the celery I also noticed a chocolate bar . . . trying to be inconspicuous. I reached for the celery and started to munch. Crunch, crunch, crunch. So different to the smooth sweet taste of chocolate melting on my tongue. But I'm being healthy, right? This is going to benefit me. Let's face it — when it comes down to a choice between celery and chocolate, who seriously is going to be happy about choosing the celery—especially after a hard day at work, an argument with a partner or friend, or just plain feeling blue? Do you feel guilty because you think that chocolate is bad for you? If so, then we have some great news for you! At last we can really know and believe that chocolate is good for us. All those negative thoughts you've had about chocolate and those guilt feelings experienced after you've enjoyed it can now be put aside. Chocolate is good for us and this book explains why.

Today there is a big emphasis on eating or avoiding particular foods to protect against some sort of disease or health condition. Take, for example, fat. We've all learned that it is important not to eat too much saturated fat. One of the consequences of doing so is that we are more likely to get heart disease. We should particularly avoid high cholesterol foods and ideally eat foods that help us lower cholesterol. Heart disease is the number-one killer in most Western countries. Many of us today have friends or know of people who've had heart bypass surgery; often at a young age. How can it be that with our modern, high-standard living we find people in their early forties with their arteries clogging up? On the other hand, we

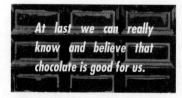

At last we can really know and believe that chocolate is good for us.

have heard stories of what's known as the French paradox; where having a glass or two of wine a day is said to protect against heart disease. People in France who drink red wine regularly seem to have a lower risk of getting heart disease even though they have a relatively high animal fat diet. There are other foods that also seem to protect against heart disease and possibly even cancer, such as soya beans and green tea.

Chocolate and Antioxidants and How the Book Came About

Of course, we've all learned that fruits and vegetables are good for us. They are good sources of fiber, vitamins, and minerals. But all these foods have another important factor in common: they are all rich in substances called "antioxidants," which protect our cells against damage and aging. Scientists have begun measuring the levels of antioxidants in more and more foods and one of the foods highest in antioxidants was, can you guess? Chocolate! In fact a small bar of chocolate had as many, if not more, antioxidants than a glass of red wine. Of course, when you find out something as exciting as this, you want to share it with friends. So, recently whenever I (Suzy) have been at a party, or social gathering, or chatting around the dinner table with friends, at a suitable time in the conversation I have let slip, "Did you know that chocolate is good for you?" Watching the expressions on people's faces was quite entertaining. The looks of disbelief, the looks that said "you must be joking!" or "don't tease us!" or "I wish it were true! I love chocolate!" I would reassure them that it was true, but still, it seemed too good to be true. (John tried this on me before we decided to write this book. My shocked expression portrayed my inner feelings of disbelief, followed by an outburst of laughter and "Come on, you can't be serious! I know that stuff makes me fat. You can't tell me that it's healthy!" However, when John explained some of the research findings to me, and I had a good look at the other fatty culprits in my diet [a weakness for shortbread and hot drinks, ice-cream, pies, and cream!], what he was saying made sense—but only, of course, if I ate chocolate in moderation!).

These findings interested me so much that, after talking to John, we decided to combine our chocolate experiences and write this book. We also decided, since I was now bubbling over with enthusiasm, that the book should have the voice of a woman—me!

To back up John's research, one day a friend told me a fascinating story. Like many women in their thirties, she had begun to put on weight after having children. She had tried different types of diets and carefully watched what she ate but still, there it was: the scales told the same story. Finally she decided, "Why bother trying? I'm going to enjoy life." One of the foods she'd been leaving out, avoiding at all costs, was chocolate. She thought, "Well, why not? Why not enjoy myself?" She found that throughout the day, when she felt like it, she would have a small piece or two of chocolate. After a while, she noticed to her amazement that she had lost weight! In fact, she felt for her age that she looked quite trim. I had to agree! However, that was not all. When she stopped eating chocolate, because she felt that surely it couldn't be good for her to be having all that sugar, she found that she began to put on weight again. This absolutely amazed her! How could it be? But, it really happened! Of course, a single story like this really doesn't prove anything, but her story stimulated our interest in the amazing benefits of chocolate.

Before you put this book down and rush to buy a month's supply of chocolate there are some important things you need to know about the chocolate story. The first is this: not all chocolate is equal! Some types of chocolate are good for you. Some chocolate is neutral. Some chocolate products are not so good for our health. This book will help you identify the types of chocolate to be avoided. We will show you how you can pick them from their labels. Second, like any good thing, you can have too much. So, how much chocolate is good for us, and when are we having too much? Perhaps a third point we should consider is that chocolate can be part of a lifestyle that gives us beauty, energy, longevity, and a reduced risk of disease. Sounds unbelievable? It's true! Chocolate can be part of enjoying life to the full; and this is what we believe chocolate symbolizes—simply enjoying life.

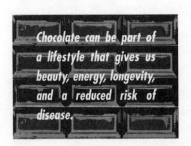

Chocolate can be part of a lifestyle that gives us beauty, energy, longevity, and a reduced risk of disease.

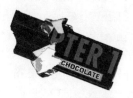

It's All in a Box of Chocolates

I've always been a big fan of chocolate, and as a child eagerly looked forward to Christmas and birthdays. Of course, the biggest chocolate festival of the year, Easter, was a mini-choc-heaven delight! I can still remember my grandmother saying to me, "Make sure you can push yourself away from the table instead of the table pushing itself away from you!" This was usually said after my sixth Easter egg and a noticeable straining of the clothes around my stomach!

Chocolate is a food that is very hard to say "no" to, but how is it made and what gives it its special seductive properties?

The Tree of Paradise? Cacao in Aztec Times

Chocolate is made from cocoa beans, which come from the Cacao tree (*Theobroma cacao*). Perhaps few chocolate eaters are aware of the extraordinary beauty of the cocoa tree, which in its native state grows in the lush jungles of Central and South America, on both sides of the equator. Imagine walking through a rain forest filled with luxuriant green trees. Occasionally a bird with breathtaking plumage flies close by, displaying a rainbow of colors in its feathers. A medium size tree with broad, dark green leaves catches your attention and you gasp in wonder at the almond-shaped fruit growing on its stems. A myriad of colors greets your eye; all different shades of reds, purples, yellows, greens, maroons, and browns. Surely, this must have been akin to the fruit Eve was tempted to eat—its colors call out to you with promise of a special food inside. It is not surprising that the Mayans and Aztecs of Mexico believed that the God of Agriculture provided the Cacao tree from Paradise and that the cocoa beans were the "food of the gods."

The Cacao tree originated in the tropical rain forests of the Amazon basin in South America and was later brought to Mexico and Costa Rica. Cacao trees are now grown in a zone 20° north and south of the equator in Brazil, Venezuela, the West Indies, Ghana, Nigeria, the Ivory Coast, Madagascar, Sri Lanka, the Philippines, Malaysia, and even Hawaii. The word "chocolate" is derived from the Aztec *xocoatl*, meaning "bitter drink." The Aztec emperor Montezuma used the beverage in his religion and the beans were used as currency. For example, we are told the value of one slave was typically 100 beans. Imagine what that would be like now . . . safes would hold chocolate bars instead of cash, and it would be considered as a sign of wealth to have a large supply of chocolate bars in your handbag!

Since ancient times, chocolate has been associated with pleasure, passion, energy, and even enhanced sexual powers. In fact the chocolate drinks prepared by the Aztecs were highly prized as a nuptial aid and not surprisingly were a favorite drink at wedding ceremonies. Tradition even has it that Montezuma was reputed to drink chocolate freely throughout the day; and always fortified himself with the beverage before entering his harem—perhaps it could be considered to be an ancient form of Viagra! Because of its renowned energy-giving properties, chocolate was also a food

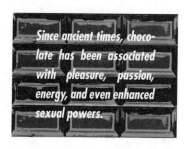

Since ancient times, chocolate has been associated with pleasure, passion, energy, and even enhanced sexual powers.

for the Aztec warriors to strengthen them on military campaigns.

Of course, the chocolate used by the Aztecs when the first Europeans reached Central America was very different to the chocolate we know today. It was a bitter brew made from cocoa beans. These fruit were put in an earthenware pot and dried over a fire. The beans were then broken between two stones and ground into a flour, just as grain would be ground to make meal for bread. This flour was transferred into another vessel, moistened gradually with water, and chilli (or "long pepper") added. The drink could then be thickened using maize meal (cornflour) to the point that it could be molded into a biscuit if necessary. In this way the chocolate could be taken as a beverage or eaten as a wafer or even as a type of porridge.

Cacao in Europe

Cacao as a beverage was brought to Europe when Columbus and Cortéz delivered beans to the King of Spain between 1502 and 1528. The Spaniards added sugar and cinnamon and heated the brew to improve the taste, and kept the beverage a secret for about a century. Cacao subsequently was introduced into France, and by 1657, into England and the North American colonies of the Dutch and English.

Growing and Harvesting Cocoa Beans

Cacao trees are now grown in plantations as well as rain forests. The tree takes about seven years to mature and produces little flower cushions that grow directly on the trunk and branches of the tree. These delicate flowers are not pollinated by bees. Instead they are pollinated by a myriad of minute flying insects which breed in the rotting jungle vegetation and live in the cool, moist conditions under the rain forest canopy. The colorful cocoa pods take about six months to ripen and yield almond-sized beans nestled in a sweet citruslike pulp. A single tree will yield about 50 to 60 pods which each contain somewhere between 20 to 40 beans.

The harvesting and the breaking open of the pods is still all done by hand—even in this age of high technology and labor-saving devices. Despite a number of attempts to design a mechanical harvester to remove cocoa pods from the tree, it has so far proved impossible. One of the reasons for this is that it's important to not damage the flower cushions which are growing nearby. Even the breaking of the pods and the extraction of the

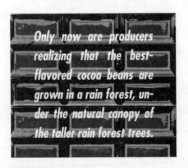

wet beans is still done by hand, even though engineers have tried for decades to develop a mechanical pod breaking and extraction machine. Cocoa is one of the few foods remaining today that are still harvested and separated totally by hand. The beans, which are 31 percent fat, 14 percent carbohydrate and 9 percent protein, are bitter because of their alkaloid content, and fermentation is necessary to develop the strong chocolate flavor.

For many years now, the majority of cocoa beans have been grown in plantations, but there is an interesting environmental twist to this practice now developing. Only now are producers realizing that the best-flavored cocoa beans are grown in a rain forest; under the natural canopy of the taller rain forest trees. The flavors of the beans grown this way are far superior to those grown in the regular plantations. Another factor coming to light is that two rainy seasons per year are ideal for the development of the pods. This has led some chocolate manufacturers to begin to actively campaign against the cutting down of rain forests and destroying the environment, and instead to encourage farmers and plantation owners to establish their cocoa trees in the rain for-

Only now are producers realizing that the best-flavored cocoa beans are grown in a rain forest, under the natural canopy of the taller rain forest trees.

est itself; and to work at preserving the total ecology of the rain forest. It is just a dream at this stage, but wouldn't it be wonderful if eating a chocolate a day could help preserve the wonderful rain forests of our planet?

That Wonderful Chocolate Flavor — How Does It Come About?

Chocolate flavor is developed in two parts: the first on the plantation by the correct fermentation of the wet beans by the grower, and the second by the processor in the factory at the roasting stage. Fermentation is achieved by leaving the beans in wooden boxes or in piles on the ground covered with banana leaves, for one to five days depending on the bean variety. The beans are then dried in the sun for another five to seven days. The dried beans are usually shipped to foreign cocoa plants where they are roasted for about 40 minutes at 100–220°C to enhance the flavor. After roasting, the beans are dehulled and the bean flesh, called *nib*, is ground to a paste now called cocoa mass or chocolate liquor which is quite bitter. Mechanical mills introduced during the industrial revolution made chocolate more available to people other than the aristocrats and nobility.

In 1828 a Dutch chemist by the name of Conrad J. van Houten developed a new type of hydraulic press with which he was able to press out about half of the cocoa butter present in the paste that was formed from grinding the beans. This left behind a brittle, cakelike residue that could be pulverized into a fine powder. Van Houten then went one step further and treated the powder with alkaline salts which improved its ability to mix with water. This process, which came to be known as "Dutching" or "alkalizing," also darkened the color of the chocolate; and at the same time lightened the flavor so that it was not quite so strong. This new process led to the manufacture of what we now know as "cocoa powder"; and revolutionized the chocolate industry. At this stage we should point out that cacao is the botanical name that refers to the tree or its pods and sometimes now also to the beans that have been fermented; whereas cocoa refers to the modern manufactured powder sold for drinking or for food manufacturing purposes.

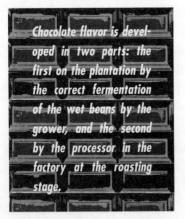

Chocolate flavor is developed in two parts: the first on the plantation by the correct fermentation of the wet beans by the grower, and the second by the processor in the factory at the roasting stage.

Have you ever tasted raw cocoa? Have you ever wanted to? I remember as a young child helping Mom cook numerous chocolate cakes, which were her specialty. One evening curiosity got the better of me and I asked Mom if I could taste some cocoa. "No," she replied, "you wouldn't like it." I didn't understand this, as I reasoned that if the mixture in the bowl containing cocoa, with sugar, eggs, flour, milk, butter, and vanilla, tasted so good all mixed up, why shouldn't cocoa taste good on its own? So when Mom's back was turned I secretly sampled the contents of the bowl, with the result that my tongue couldn't cope with the subtle flavors of raw cocoa and my face and stomach convulsed with distaste.

Perfecting the Technique

The important question is: how is cocoa, that brown, dirtlike substance, turned into a food which few people can resist? Well, it seems that not long after van Houten's process became known, one of the chocolate manufacturers hit on the idea of melting the cocoa butter and combining it with a blend of the ground cocoa beans and sugar. The resulting mixture was a smooth and workable pastelike material that enabled additional sugar to be added without becoming gritty. This new pastelike material could be poured into molds and cast, and this became the first eating chocolate.

Sugar and milk solids were added to the cocoa solids to produce milk chocolate in the Swiss process introduced by Henri Nestlé in 1875. The refining of this mixture by grinding between rollers for up to 72 hours reduced the particles to a mere dozen or so microns in size, giving this chocolate the smooth-mouth feel we have come to expect from quality chocolate.

Another development in the manufacture of modern chocolate soon followed, again in Switzerland. In 1880 the conching machine was invented by a Swiss chocolatier, Rodolfe Lindt. The function of this machine is to stir the liquid chocolate gently over a period of time. It is during this process that the final flavors of the chocolate are developed. Any residual bitterness is removed. Conched chocolates typically are described as being less harsh and having a more balanced flavor profile. The conching process is the final stage in the art of making chocolate and important changes in the flavor are produced during this process. Certain volatile flavors are lost; while at the same time other flavors are added; for example, vanilla, mint, cloves, or cinnamon. The use of vanilla dates back to the days of the Aztecs, who also added this particular plant extract to their drink. Today pure vanilla extract is used for the best quality chocolates, but cheaper, mass-produced chocolates are more likely to contain the synthetic flavor known as vanillin.

Different Ingredients for Different Chocolates

Have you ever looked at the ingredients list on a chocolate wrapper? Have you ever wondered what the recipes are for different types of chocolate? And how can white chocolate be called "chocolate" when it isn't brown? Well, a quality dark chocolate recipe typically would consist of about 30 percent sugar, which has been finely ground, about 70 percent cocoa liquor, which would include about 30 percent cocoa butter, and a small amount of lecithin and pure vanilla extract; perhaps around 1 percent in total. Mass-produced milk chocolate is typically made with around 10 percent cocoa mass, 23 percent cocoa butter, 40 percent sugar, and about 26 percent milk solids, as well as small amounts of emulsifiers and flavors. White chocolate has no cocoa solids and is made instead from the cocoa butter by itself, with added sugar, milk, flavoring, and emulsifiers such as lecithin. Of course, white chocolate doesn't have the same depth of flavor as milk chocolate or plain chocolate, but it still has the lovely, rich, and creamy mouth feel of normal chocolate.

Because cocoa liquor is so expensive, there is a tendency to substitute cheaper ingredients, and this can include sugar. It's much cheaper to add more sugar to the chocolate and reduce the amount of cocoa liquor. Another way to reduce the cost of chocolate manufacture is to use hardened vegetable fats instead of cocoa butter. We shall see in Chapter 5 that these types of chocolates have totally different health properties.

Another type of chocolate is couverture. This is a high quality chocolate used mainly for coatings and in baking. How many times have you intended to make chocolate chip cookies, but those small mounds of smooth sweetness made it irresistible to take just one, or two, then three? Before you know it, the packet is gone and the butter, sugar, and flour are sitting forlornly on the bench beside the mixing bowl. Couvertures have a higher percentage of cocoa butter, and this enables them to form very thin coatings.

Chocolate can be poured into different molds, and formed into bars and different shapes. It can be used to coat products such as muesli bars, nuts (such as almonds, hazelnuts, brazil nuts, and peanuts), and dried fruit such as sultanas and raisins. On the other hand, nuts and fruit are often added to chocolate; for example a Fruit and Nut milk chocolate. Other sweet fillings can be coated with chocolate and these are often found in the well-known box of chocolates. In fact, a box of chocolates is one of the traditional Western dating gifts, along with a bunch of fresh flowers—the sure way to any girl's heart! And what honeymoon suite would be the same without a beautifully arranged box of complimentary chocolates? With mouth-watering fillings made from different fruit creams and liqueurs (such as cherries, cumquats or peaches, pears, apricots, and oranges), few people find a box of chocolates easy to resist! Additional fillings include truffles laced with champagne, chunks of stem ginger and exotic toffees. Of course, enjoying a box of chocolates doesn't have to be restricted to dating and honeymoons.

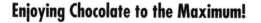

Enjoying Chocolate to the Maximum!

To the chocolate connoisseur, even eating chocolate is an art. Much like wine tasting and tasting a fine coffee, it can be a sensual experience. It's been suggested that to really enjoy chocolate it should be allowed to come to a room temperature of around 66–77°F. For a plain chocolate, tasting involves placing the chocolate in your mouth for a few moments to just enjoy the primary flavors and aromas of the chocolate, and then, as you bite on

the chocolate, chewing it slowly a few times, to release the secondary aromas. Then, let the chocolate just rest against the roof and sides of your
mouth and tongue so that you experience the full
range of flavors, and as the chocolate melts enjoy
the lingering taste in your mouth. The experts say
chocolate should be eaten slowly, in small
amounts, and enjoyed. It is a food that brings so
much pleasure when eaten correctly.

A filled chocolate is perhaps eaten a little differ-
ently. In this case the experts suggest that the
chocolate be allowed to sit in your mouth for a few
moments; again to release the primary flavors and
aromas. It should then be chewed up to five times
to mix the chocolate and the filling, then allow this
mixture to melt slowly so that you experience a new
range of the flavors produced by the mingling of the
chocolate and its filling. Again you must allow the
taste to linger in the mouth before swallowing. We
find chocolate is an ideal way to finish a meal, but
generally speaking chocolate and wine do not mix.
This may be surprising to
you, but the reason given is
that the lingering intensity
of the chocolate can com-
pete with the flavor and
aroma of the wine.

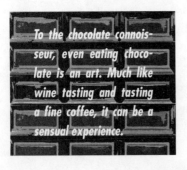

To the chocolate connois-
seur, even eating choco-
late is an art. Much like
wine tasting and tasting
a fine coffee, it can be a
sensual experience.

Making individual chocolates can be another form of art. How many times have you looked in amazement at the different shapes and swirls and patterns that have been used to decorate chocolate? Chocolates can have a beauty all of their own, and there is abundant skill used to create the shapes and design of the different forms of chocolate. There are also the chocolate wrappings. The chocolates themselves are visual and edible art and the wrappings are art to delight the eye. The different patterns, the colors, the types of material again can bring so much pleasure. They offer a whole new area of creativity for the artist-designer. They convey messages of enjoyment, of love, affection, endearment, and having fun. Chocolate is truly a food of Paradise.

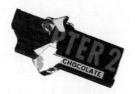

The Best Food for Mood

How do you feel after you've just taken that first bite into a luscious piece of chocolate? The sweet taste glides over your tongue and the chocolate melts slowly from the warmth of your mouth. Feelings of euphoria well up deep inside you as you swallow and sigh with contentment. Have you wondered whether that feeling came from the chocolate, or was it just your body's reaction to relaxing and having a break?

That Euphoric Effect . . .

One of the reasons we enjoy chocolate so much is because it produces the effect of euphoria after we begin to eat it. A reason for this is that chocolate contains a phytochemical called phenylethylamine (PEA). This particular substance belongs to a group of chemicals known as endorphins. These have a stimulating effect on the brain. When released into the bloodstream, endorphin-like chemicals lift the mood. They create a positive energy and feelings ranging from happiness to euphoria. These are similar to the feelings known as a "runner's high." It can create the effect of increasing our energy and apparent mental alertness.

When I was at college, chocolate was the most sought-after study food. People would go in groups to the nearest supermarket and raid the shelves for all-night feasts. When that supply was exhausted, the college canteen was hit with a barrage of chocolate-craving students, usually around 11 P.M. after the final basketball game (when we pretended to study). My friends and I would often join this motley crowd and grab as much chocolate as we could, then go back to the dorm and set up "chocolate picnics" to help us through another long night with the books. If any of the kids from the nearby schools wanted money for fund-raising, all they had to do was turn up at the girls' dorm and announce that they were selling chocolates, and they would be stampeded by females waving money at them! Sometimes I think it might have been a bit daunting for those younger men.

John quotes a study from two New York psychoanalysts who were treating a group of "love addicted" women some years ago. These psychoanalysts found that the women produced large amounts of PEA in the brain. When the women's infatuation stopped, so did the production of PEA. All of us at some time or another have experienced falling in love. It may have been at school, or at college, or later in life. It is the most wonderful event; highlighted perhaps by the feelings of pleasure that we experience just by being in the presence of the one we love. Interestingly, eating chocolate can produce the same feelings of pleasure. This gives rise to the many sayings (mainly by women!) along the lines that chocolate is more satisfying than sex. When we are in love, our brain re-

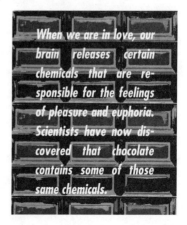

When we are in love, our brain releases certain chemicals that are responsible for the feelings of pleasure and euphoria. Scientists have now discovered that chocolate contains some of those same chemicals.

leases certain chemicals which are responsible for the feelings of pleasure and euphoria that we enjoy. Scientists have now discovered that chocolate contains some of those same chemicals; which confirms that the pleasurable experiences we enjoy from eating chocolate are in fact real. Not surprisingly chocolate is closely associated with romance and close friendship.

When PEA is produced by brain tissue, it is distributed within the central nervous system. Several studies have suggested that PEA is an important modulator of mood, and that when we do not have enough PEA in our brain we experience the illness of depression. It has been shown that people suffering severe depression have very low levels of PEA in their body. On the other hand, chocolate contains substantial levels of PEA; with levels ranging from about 0.4 up to 6.6 micrograms per gram of chocolate. Of course, chocolate is not the only food that contains PEA. Substantially greater quantities are found in common foods such as cheeses, and in certain sausages.

Chocolate Can Help PMS

Many people experience intense cravings for chocolate and women in particular can find that they are craving chocolate just before and during their period. In fact, a survey about food cravings administered to undergraduates at a university documented chocolate as the most frequently mentioned craved substance among women. Thirty-two percent of women reported an association with the menstrual cycle. Other foods craved at this time included pleasant tasting, sweet, high-fat foods. There is no doubt that these cravings are real. In the case of chocolate, some experts contend that the cravings may be an attempt to self-regulate brain PEA levels and mood. So, as Karen Scalf Linamen writes in the title of her bestselling book for women: *Just Hand Over the Chocolate and No One Will Get Hurt!*

Chocolate often makes us feel better when we're feeling blue or upset. Forget the Hallmark cards that say "I'm sorry," just buy me a box of fine chocolates and all will be forgiven! One survey of women found that 68 percent of women at some time craved chocolate; and 50 percent of women would choose chocolate in preference to making love! Twenty-two percent were more likely than men to choose chocolate as a mood elevator. A prominent young actress is quoted to have said that "Sex is good, but chocolate with sex is even better!" When women crave chocolate around the time of their periods, eating chocolate can act as a mood elevator and help to alleviate the pain and depression associated with menstruation. The following true experience illustrates this.

Driving home from work one afternoon my husband, whom I just married, asked me how my day was. "Okay," I replied shortly. This was followed by a long silence. My husband and I usually talk nonstop on the drive home, sharing our workday experiences. He must have perceived that things were different that day and asked me what was wrong—was it something he had said?

"No, and nothing," was again my barely audible reply.

Undeterred by this apparent lack of enthusiasm, my husband persisted by asking, "Are you sure?"

The lion inside me wanted to roar as yet another knife-stabbing pain seared through the lower half of my body. "I'll be fine, honey," I said in measured breaths, "if you'll just buy me a chocolate bar."

So he did.

About a month later we were in a local shopping center when my husband rather tentatively pointed out to me, "Honey, there's a pile of family-size chocolate blocks over there, if you'd like some."

There are many other ways chocolate can affect our mood. For example, the smell of chocolate has been found to slow down brain waves, making us feel calm. Most of the time our brains are dominated by what are called "beta waves" (the normal waking frequency). When our brain activity slows to alpha waves, we experience a pleasant feeling of calm but alert relaxation. Also, because most of us find eating chocolate so pleasurable, we release endorphins. These are also released in the brain during times of other pleasurable activities, such as during sex. These endorphins have similar pharmacological actions as morphine, acting as pain relievers and giving us a sense of well-being.

Another fascinating reason we women may crave chocolate just before menstruation is the body's intuitive reaction to supplement its requirement for magnesium. Magnesium is an important element which we mention

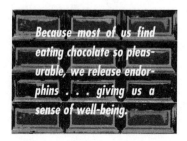

Because most of us find eating chocolate so pleasurable, we release endorphins . . . giving us a sense of well-being.

in a later chapter and is associated with calcium to make healthy bones and teeth. However, medical researchers have now found that magnesium deficiency may contribute to the symptoms of premenstrual syndrome (PMS). It is also known that stress stimulates the increased excretion of magnesium from our body. Magnesium deficiency results in selective depletion of central nervous system levels of dopamine, a neurotransmitter that transmits signals of euphoria and satisfaction. Dopamine also plays an important role in the brain in balancing out another neurotransmitter found in the central nervous system called "serotonin." Eating a lot of sweet, high-carbohydrate foods can stimulate the brain to produce high levels of serotonin. However, if these elevated levels of serotonin are unopposed by dopamine, then we may experience the primary symptoms of PMS. Getting extra magnesium by eating chocolate can help restore dopamine levels to balance the serotonin and thereby reduce PMS.

Chocolate and cocoa powder both contain high concentrations of magnesium, which women's bodies need at this time. Therefore, we should not feel guilty about our chocolate cravings at that time of the month. But this is no excuse to get carried away with overeating chocolate. Remember, the ideal maximum intake of chocolate is about 2 ounces a day, that is, an average size chocolate bar. This is also why in a chapter later on we talk about what other healthy ways we can ensure that we get ample amounts of magnesium and the other important nutrients.

There is also another intriguing side to the serotonin story. Low levels of serotonin in the brain have also been associated with depression and a craving for carbohydrates, including chocolate. It has been recently discovered that sunlight entering our eyes during the day stimulates the production of serotonin in the brain. This does not mean that we need to look directly at the sun! To do so can cause serious eye problems. When we expose our eyes to insufficient bright light during the day, by continually working indoors, particularly in winter time, this can lead to decreased levels of serotonin. In the past, this type of depression has often been referred to as "winter blues." If we find that we are developing a carbohydrate craving and perhaps feeling depressed, it may be time to take stock as to whether or not we are getting sufficient daylight exposure in our daily routine.

John came across findings from researchers at Columbia University who

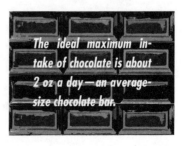

The ideal maximum intake of chocolate is about 2 oz a day—an average-size chocolate bar.

discovered that exposing patients with severe carbohydrate cravings to two and a half thousand lux of light (this is, light about five times the intensity of the usual indoor illumination) for two hours in the morning brought a complete remission from both depression and carbohydrate craving in half the patients treated; with the other half showing definite improvement. The researchers found that light in the morning is more effective than light later in the day.

While scientists are still learning about the importance of daylight and sunlight exposure for our well-being, getting up that little bit extra in the morning to enable an early morning walk before work, and avoiding wearing sunglasses on days when it isn't really necessary, and getting out of the office into the outdoors at lunch time can complement the benefits that we can get from eating chocolate.

Chocolate Is Not an Illegal Substance!

In 1996, researchers at the Neuroscientists Institute in San Diego, California, published a fascinating paper in the prestigious science journal *Nature*, which was called "Brain Cannabinoids in Chocolate." Neurons in our brain produce and release a chemical which is called "anandamide" which literally means "internal bliss." This chemical is an endogenous brain lipoprotein which binds to and activates cannabinoid receptors within the brain. This results in a psychoactive effect of heightened sensitivity and euphoria which is similar to the reported effects of psychoactive cannabinoid drugs such as marijuana. Anandamide can increase the activity of dopamine and other neurochemicals found in the brain. It appears that chocolate contains chemicals relating to anandamide which extend its activity in the brain and therefore extend the consequential effects of well-being.

Not long after this research was published, a Belgian lawyer attempted to have his client cleared of a charge of smoking and dealing in marijuana by suggesting that the accused had supposedly eaten a massive amount of chocolate which contained cannabinoid mimics. According to the lawyer these were the cause of the positive cannabinoid test. This claim was subsequently investigated by scientists. The study, which was published in the March 2000 issue of the *International Journal of Legal Medicine*, showed that the chocolate could not be responsible for the positive cannabinoid test and as a result the lawyer's claim could be refuted and the accused was convicted. Before we get too worried, we need to remember that a 130 lb woman would need to eat more than 22 lbs of chocolate to get a "buzz."

The Stimulants Found in Chocolate

One compound in chocolate that we hear more about is caffeine, the stimulant that is also found in coffee, tea, and cola drinks. Caffeine interacts with neuromodulators in the brain (causing a greater sense of alertness) and catalyses other compounds from the adrenal gland which mildly stimulate the central nervous system. High levels of caffeine in the diet can make children hyperactive or anxious and, in adults who are under stress, caffeine may cause the blood pressure to rise even further. However, what we need to remember is that the levels of caffeine in chocolate are relatively low. Coffee, tea, and cola drinks are by far the main sources of caffeine in the diet. In fact, a cup of hot chocolate contains about the same amount of caffeine as a cup of decaffeinated coffee. A 20 g (just over ½ oz) serve of milk chocolate would contain only about 4 milligrams of caffeine compared to 60–90 milligrams of caffeine in the average cup of coffee, and low levels of caffeine, less than 20 milligrams, do not appear to have a detectable effect on the body. Even a 50 g (2 oz) dark chocolate bar would contain only around 38 milligrams of caffeine, which would be less than the caffeine in a cup of tea or the average standard cola drink.

Of course, chocolate also contains other weaker stimulants such as theobromine. This natural substance is a very mild heart stimulant but it also has the properties of being a smooth muscle relaxant and a vasodilator. It can actually help in a very mild way to lower blood pressure.

We've all heard the saying "Oh no! Not death by chocolate!" when someone brings a large plate of chocolate into the room. Of course, death by chocolate is very unlikely. I saw in a restaurant once a dish titled Death by Chocolate, and for my eighteenth birthday party we had a huge death-by-chocolate feast. Everything on the menu was chocolate or chocolate-based. The only effect we felt from so much indulgence was mild nausea and a lot of energy to burn off! It was awhile, however, before I ate anything chocolate again!

We should not, however, feed our favorite pets chocolate. Dogs and cats can become quite ill from eating chocolate. It seems that theobromine has a much more dramatic effect on the heart rate of these animals. Therefore it is, theoretically, possible to kill these animals by giving them large quantities of

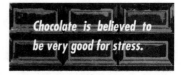
Chocolate is believed to be very good for stress.

chocolate. The effect on humans is quite different. In a similar way a funnel-web spider bite can be deadly to humans, whereas our cats and dogs are immune to the venom of this spider.

While chocolate contains stimulants such as caffeine and theobromine, believe it or not, chocolate is believed to be very good for stress. This is thought to be because it contains another substance called valeric acid which is a relaxant and tranquilizer. We can see that chocolate is an amazing food and a natural blend of compounds that make us feel good. As M. Roach wrote in her article "More Reasons to Love Chocolate" (*New Woman*, February 1989, page 135): "caviar is exquisite, but people don't declare their love with 10 pound heart-shaped boxes of it . . . no one makes 3 A.M. runs to the 7–11 for butterscotch, but chocolate . . . chocolate inspires a passion normally reserved for things grander than food."

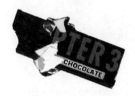

Why Chocolate Is a Health Food

Chocolate—a health food? It sounds too good to be true, doesn't it? Surely, how can anything that sweet and tasting . . . so, so . . . nice be a health food? If someone told us that chocolate was a health food, most of us would probably be skeptical. It goes against everything that we've ever been taught about chocolate; like it makes you fat, gives you pimples, and the dentist will be seeing you quite often to fill in the tooth cavities. A health food store would be the last place anyone would think of looking for chocolate. How could something so sweet and delicious be healthy? It just doesn't seem to fit into the image of things found there. On the contrary, we'd expect to find things like organic fruits and vegetables, or perhaps an array of herbal teas.

What Is a Health Food?

Many of us think of health foods in terms of high fiber breakfast cereals or whole-meal breads with lots of cracked wheat and other whole grains in them. Indeed, if we went into the average health food store what would we see there? There would be a display of organically grown dried fruits, many of them without preservatives, and packets of nuts such as almonds, cashews, brazil nuts, and walnuts. We would see exotic whole-grain breads, packets of the less common grains such as millet and buckwheat, food supplements such as brewer's yeast and lecithin, packets of linseed, sunflower seeds and pepitas, as well as cold pressed oils such as linseed and macadamia. There would be muesli bars, sweetened perhaps with honey and containing all sorts of seeds (including hemp seeds). We might even see exotic things like hemp pasta and sprouted hemp seed bread. But would we expect to find chocolate? Not likely. But there would be carob. We would find carob-coated peanuts and sultanas, carob bars and maybe even little carob sweets. But why not chocolate?

In fact, if we found regular chocolate in a health food store many of us would perhaps doubt the integrity of the proprietor. We would probably find chocolate's well-known substitute carob, which has been shown to many of us as the healthier alternative to chocolate. But think about it—what is a health food? Perhaps the first picture that comes to mind is that it's a whole food. It is a food that has close to all the nutrition that it would have if we ate it fresh in the field. In other words, it has had minimum processing. For example, stone-ground whole-meal flour is simply ground up whole wheat. On the other hand, the white flour that is the most commonly sold in the supermarket and that is used for making the standard white bread has been refined to make it white. In the refining process the bran and the germ are removed and along with them the important nutrients they contain, such as fiber, potassium, and magnesium. So we do not usually find white bread in a health food shop.

Let us now think about some of the other things we find in health food shops, such as brewer's yeast and cold pressed lin-

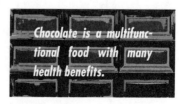

Chocolate is a multifunctional food with many health benefits.

seed oil. These foods are found there because they supply particular functional properties. The brewer's yeast may be a source of chromium and B vitamins. The cold pressed linseed oil (or flaxseed oil) supplies us with the omega 3 fatty acids. These foods are not usually eaten by themselves but are used to supplement our diet with the nutrients that are often missing in our modern processed foods. Generally speaking, for a healthy diet we need a variety of foods and for optimum health we need a variety of foods that deliver a range of different types of nutrients. That is, they are rich sources of fiber, minerals, or antioxidants and vitamins. This is where chocolate fits in. As you progress through this book you will find that chocolate has many aspects to its nutrition. In other words, it is a multifunctional food with many health benefits.

Chocolate and Minerals

Cocoa is almost unique in being a veritable storehouse of minerals. Cocoa and chocolate perhaps contain more minerals than any other food. According to the food analysis tables, cocoa contains more iron than any other vegetable. The level of iron in cocoa powder is typically 14 milligrams per 100 g (about 3½ oz). Cocoa is also an excellent source of potassium and phosphorus as well as being good sources of zinc, copper, and manganese, which are important trace elements that our bodies need. In fact, researchers and dieticians have found that chocolate is a major source of dietary copper, in the North American diet. Copper is now believed to be another trace mineral with an important role in preventing heart disease. Researchers have also found that the iron present in cocoa powder is 93 percent usable, and 85 percent of the phosphorus is reported to be in a form that the body can use as a nutrient.

Some nutritionists have raised questions about a compound called oxalic acid which is found in small amounts in chocolate. Oxalic acid can combine with minerals such as iron and calcium in a way which makes these elements not available to the body. However, we have already noted that the iron in chocolate is highly bioavailable, indicating that this form of oxalate does not adversely affect this mineral. In fact, when many common foods were analyzed for their oxalic acid content, it was found that foods such as spinach, tea, beetroot, and even peanuts actually contained more oxalate than chocolate.

Of course, there's another important side to the mineral story. Most minerals, when taken into the body, are stored for use at just the right time.

Some nutrition authorities are concerned about people taking supplements with specific minerals in them which may upset the body's natural balance. Taking too much of one mineral can cause a depletion in another mineral. If you're taking mineral supplements on a regular basis and have concerns about mineral depletion, it's perhaps best to talk to your doctor. It seems that one of the best ways we can get our minerals is to get them naturally from foods that are good sources. Chocolate contains minerals such as magnesium, copper, iron, potassium, chromium, zinc, and manganese. It really can be considered a natural mineral supplement!

Chocolate—Low in Sodium, High in Potassium

The other really good thing about chocolate is that many chocolates are low in sodium (salt), which is one mineral that we tend to get too much of in our modern, Western diets. So in this regard we can see that eating chocolate is a wonderful way to get our minerals naturally; perhaps *better* than taking a mineral supplement.

When we study the nutritional attributes of chocolate more closely, one of the first things we discover is that chocolate is an excellent source of potassium. In fact chocolate contains more than one and a half times as much potassium as whole-meal bread, and cocoa powder contains up to ten times as much! Why is potassium important in our diet? Potassium is perhaps one of the most over-looked factors in health. It is one of the important elements that we get in vegetables, whole grains, and particularly bran. One reason why whole foods are so important is that they have a higher level of potassium than sodium, whereas most processed foods have a much higher level of sodium than potassium. Whole-meal wheat flour, for example, has 63 times as much potassium as sodium; whereas commercial whole-meal bread, which contains added salt, has nearly twice as much sodium as potassium. In other words, we have changed the natural ratio around by a factor of around 110 times. If we take the popular break-fast cereal cornflakes with its added salt, it con-tains nearly 12 times more sodium than potassium. By contrast, in natural corn we find there is 180 times more potassium than sodium. What does this mean? It means that today in our Western diet, with all the

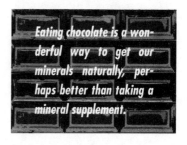

Eating chocolate is a wonderful way to get our minerals naturally, perhaps better than taking a mineral supplement.

added salt in our processed foods, we are getting far more sodium than we should be for good health.

Our hormone production glands and kidney systems are designed to conserve water and sodium while excreting potassium. That is, our body is designed for a relatively high potassium intake, and the operation of many cellular functions within the human body are maintained by a delicate balance between sodium and potassium. For optimum health we need to preserve that balance by avoiding adding too much salt to our diet.

When there is a chronic excess of salt, which is possible whenever our diet is high in processed food, this subtle distortion resulting from the high sodium diet means that our required amounts for dietary potassium are now much higher. Other substances in the diet can also exacerbate the potassium problem. Alcohol, for example, can contribute to increased potassium deficiency in that it encourages the urinary secretion of potassium. This is where chocolate and cocoa can come in as important foods to restore the potassium balance. Chocolate and cocoa, as we have seen, are not only excellent sources of potassium but they contain no added salt. By regularly having some chocolate in our diet we can help counteract some of the imbalances caused by much of the processed foods that many of us tend to eat today.

So why is potassium so important for health? Well, potassium is necessary for the normal growth and development of the body, and works with sodium to normalize the muscular system and to regulate the body's water balance. In regard to the muscular system, potassium plays a role in stimulating the nerve impulses required for muscle contraction and, together with calcium, regulates the neuro-muscular activity.

Potassium is also involved in the regulation of oxygen levels in the brain. It assists in the conversion of glucose to glycogen, the form of energy in which glucose is stored in the liver and muscles. The early indications of potassium deficiency are general muscle weakness, or tiredness. To maximize muscle strength and overall energy, it is important to reduce our salt intake and increase the levels of potassium available in our body. Low levels of potassium in the diet may contribute to the effects of chronic fatigue syndrome. One research team, led by Dr. Richard Burnett at a large Australian teaching hospital, has found that patients with chronic fatigue syndrome (CFS) have sig-

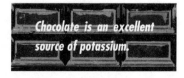

Chocolate is an excellent source of potassium.

nificantly lower levels of total body potassium than a matched control sample of people.

Potassium deficiency may also lead to various nervous disorders, including insomnia. If you have trouble sleeping, it's worth increasing your potassium intake while decreasing your sodium intake. Older people may experience dry skin from too little potassium, while adolescents may develop acne.

Diabetes may be one disease indirectly linked to the potassium/sodium imbalance. Diabetic patients are commonly deficient in potassium. Including some chocolate in the diet can be an excellent way to boost potassium levels even for diabetics. In a later chapter, we will see that chocolate, despite the common perception, is actually a food that can be eaten in moderation quite safely by most diabetics. Of course, chocolate is not the only way to get potassium. We should include in our diet lots of fresh fruits and vegetables and whole grains, and at the same time minimize the amount of processed foods that we include in the diet. Having a diet balanced in whole foods, including fish, legumes, and soy is one of the best ways of reducing the risk of developing diabetes.

Magnesium and Calcium Found in Chocolate

Chocolate is also an excellent source of two other important elements for health: calcium and magnesium. We hear a lot about calcium in the media and how it is important for healthy teeth and bones to have adequate calcium in the diet. Today we see milks and soy beverages fortified with calcium as well as calcium-fortified breakfast cereals and other foods. We think of milk and dairy products as excellent sources of calcium, but did you know that cocoa powder contains more calcium than whole milk? Of course, cocoa is a powder and we would not use as much at a serving compared to milk. If you don't drink milk, milk chocolate can be a particularly important source of calcium in the diet.

When calcium occurs naturally in foods it usually occurs with its important co-nutrient magnesium. This is another area where chocolate can play an important part in our health. Cocoa is one of the richest sources of magnesium. In fact, it has more than eight times as much as whole-meal bread. Calcium and magnesium work together. Magnesium regulates the amount of calcium that enters cells

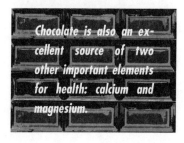

Chocolate is also an excellent source of two other important elements for health: calcium and magnesium.

and is necessary for the prevention of osteoporosis. A deficiency of magnesium can induce muscle spasms and cramps, as well as heartbeat abnormalities. Magnesium is now believed to be a very important heart protection factor.

The best sources of magnesium are the green leafy vegetables, whole-grain foods, and nuts in particular. And since cocoa powder has one of the highest levels of magnesium, a hot chocolate drink at bedtime can also be a daily heart protecting tonic.

Chocolate and cocoa drinks are excellent sources of other important minerals, too, such as iron and phosphorus, zinc, and copper. These minerals play an important role in our health. They are exactly the same minerals that we associate with the traditional health foods of whole-grains and green leafy vegetables. So, for this reason alone we could consider chocolate a health food as it is such a rich source of these nutrients. But the story doesn't end there. Not by a long way! One set of nutrients we have not talked about are the polyphenolic antioxidants that are found in red wines and green tea and also in chocolate. In fact, as we shall see, choco-

> *Chocolate and cocoa drinks are excellent sources of other important minerals, too, such as iron and phosphorus, zinc, and copper.*

late contains similar levels of these antioxidants to red wine. These health-protecting compounds are so important that we have devoted the next chapter of this book to these anti-aging nutrients that are found in chocolate.

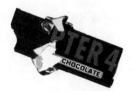

Chocolate—The Best Thing Since Red Wine

If there is one food that has captured our attention and inspired imagination as much as chocolate, it has to be wine. Wine has been associated with love and romance for centuries. It is even traditional in some wedding ceremonies for the couple to have a small drink with the officiating priest. Care needs to be taken, however, that you don't drink too much . . . you want to end up marrying the right man, after all! Wine is also associated with fine dining and for several years now there's been much talk about the health benefits of red wine. Well, now scientists have discovered that chocolate may be as good as, or even better than, red wine!

The French Paradox

Red wine is the central ingredient in a phenomenon—an apparent contradiction—known as the French paradox. It was discovered when researchers were studying heart disease in France. It was noticed that although the French people in general had a high intake of saturated fat, they reportedly had a lower incidence of heart disease than one would expect from the level of fat in their diet.

Scientists were baffled by this, as the harmful effects of a diet high in saturated fat were all too well known. However, they also noticed that French people were among the highest consumers of wine in the world. This then raised the question—was there a connection between wine drinking and protection against the effects of a high saturated fat diet? As the scientists investigated further they found that it was particularly red wine that seemed to confer this protective effect. Red wine was found to be characteristically different from

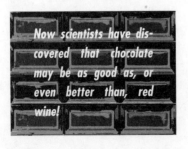

Now scientists have discovered that chocolate may be as good as, or even better than, red wine!

white wine in that red wine had very high levels of compounds known as flavonoids; and in particular a class of flavonoids known as "polyphenolics." These are naturally occurring compounds that are often responsible for the dark colors in foods like dark grape juice and tea. As research continued, scientists found that these polyphenolic compounds were very potent antioxidants; and that the antioxidant function appeared to be protecting the cholesterol in the high fat diet from oxidation, and exerting its harmful artery clogging (atherogenic) effects on the body. A glass of wine a day seemed to be sufficient to exert a measurable protective effect. This is why some doctors say that a glass of red wine a day is good for your heart.

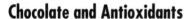

Chocolate and Antioxidants

About the same time as the studies into the health benefits of red wine were going on, other researchers were finding that drinking green tea seemed to confer a protective effect against cancer. Populations in China and Japan who drank large quantities of green tea were observed to have much lower rates of cancer. Again, scientists found that green tea contained high levels of polyphenolic antioxidant compounds. These important separate findings catalyzed intense interest in the natural antioxidants that are in our diet. As more foods were studied, one food group emerged as being an outstanding source of polyphenolic type antioxidant compounds. These were (can you guess?) chocolate and cocoa products. In fact, it was found that a 40 g (1½ oz) bar of milk chocolate contained about the same level of polyphenolic antioxidants as a glass of red wine.

To put this in perspective, the antioxidant activity of a 150 ml (about 5 fl. oz) glass of red wine is roughly equivalent to that of 12 glasses of white wine, or two cups of tea, or four apples, or five servings of onions, or three glasses of blackcurrant juice, or three 500 ml (about 16 fl. oz) glasses of beer, or seven glasses of orange juice, or 20 glasses of long-life apple juice. Many fruits and vegetables are good sources of natural polyphenolic antioxidants but none of them come near the levels that are found in the cocoa bean or tea. In terms of measurements, a 150 ml (5 fl. oz) glass of red wine or a 40 g (1½ oz) bar of milk chocolate contains about 200 milligrams of standard polyphenols. A cup of hot chocolate containing two tablespoons (or

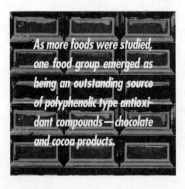

As more foods were studied, one food group emerged as being an outstanding source of polyphenolic type antioxidant compounds—chocolate and cocoa products.

about 7.3 g) of cocoa would have around 145 milligrams of polyphenols. The antioxidant properties of chocolate should come as no surprise to us. It has been known for decades that chocolate seems to keep almost indefinitely, at least for several years, yet chocolate contains high levels of fat. During that time the fat does not go rancid; that is, it does not oxidize. It turns out that chocolate contains these natural antioxidants that protect the fat during this storage time.

This protective quality has made chocolate an ideal food for soldiers. In some cases during the Second World War, U.S. troops were rationed three chocolate bars per day during heavy combat as their sole source of nourishment. The caffeine and high sugar concentration in chocolate provided a good source of rapidly absorbed energy. Its high fat content provided a sustained energy source. It now seems that the flavonoids prevented the product from "going off." This enabled it to be carried for a long period of time.

This reminds me of an incident which occurred on my fifth birthday. We had a treasure hunt where Mom creatively hid a number of chocolate frogs. About a year later I was playing outside and found a chocolate frog, wrapper still intact. Unfortunately, Mom wouldn't let me eat it as it had been hidden in the sandpit, a favorite place for all the neighborhood cats to meet!

Another aspect that has emerged from the antioxidant research is that the chocolate made from the fermented cocoa beans seems to have higher levels of polyphenolics than in the straight beans. This means that the quality chocolates made from the fermented cocoa beans are going to be superior in terms of health benefits to the cocoa products that are made by simply grinding the straight cocoa beans, as used in some of the cheaper cocoa products—another example of the old adage that you get what you pay for. It now appears that during the fermentation process certain of the polyphenol-type flavonoids are polymerized—that is, they combine to form larger molecules, and that these larger molecules have strikingly better antioxidant properties.

Why Are Antioxidants Good?

"Antioxidants" is now a catchword of the new millennium. Everyone from cosmetic companies to the medical profession is aware of the advantages of antioxidants, and with good reason—antioxidants are believed to play a very important role in helping to slow the aging process and prevent cancer and heart disease.

We need to ensure that we have an ample supply of antioxidants in our diet to deal with the extra free radicals in our environment. Free radicals are produced by the natural biochemical reactions that occur in our bodies when we are exposed to the air we breathe (cigarette smoke, air pollution), the food and water we consume, and even sunlight. Because free radicals are compounds with at least one odd or unpaired electron, this makes them unstable and very reactive. They can damage cells and tissues, causing adverse effects on the functioning of our bodies. Antioxidants such as vitamin C, vitamin E, and polyphenols can react with free radicals and protect the health-giving processes in our body.

The cosmetic section in any department store or exclusive salon contains display shelves devoted to lotions saturated with vitamin E, which we are told will help delay premature aging of the skin. We are also told from an early age that taking vitamin C is a natural way to help stop colds developing in winter. So, generally speaking, we are aware of the benefits these vitamins can bring us. Dr. Ivor Dreosti from the Australian Commonwealth Scientific and Industrial Research Organization, writing in

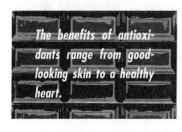

The benefits of antioxidants range from good-looking skin to a healthy heart.

2000 in the journal *Nutrition*, points out that some polyphenolic antioxidants are actually more potent than vitamin C or vitamin E. Polyphenols isolated from water extracts of green tea have been shown in animal studies to afford protection against chemically induced cancer in the lung, stomach, esophagus, duodenum, pancreas, and liver.

The High Levels of Antioxidants in Chocolate

John refers to two reports published in the *Journal of Agriculture and Food Chemistry* in 1999, showing that careful chemical analysis by scientists from the Department of Nutrition at the University of California, Davis, found that the antioxidant level in chocolate is actually higher than in tea. One of the reasons for this is that the earlier measurements underestimated the content of polyphenolics in chocolate. This was because the early methods of analysis only measured the small

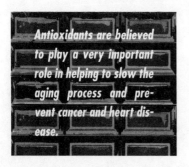

Antioxidants are believed to play a very important role in helping to slow the aging process and prevent cancer and heart disease.

molecule types of polyphenols in chocolate. In fermented cocoa products there are also large molecule type polyphenols known as procyanidins. There is now evidence that the procyanidins are 15 to 30 times more effective at quenching oxygen type free radicals than are the smaller polyphenols found in green tea. It is thought that because these large compounds are not absorbed, they could exert their antioxidant activity within the digestive tract and protect fats and proteins and carbohydrates from oxidative damage during digestion. They may even spare other soluble antioxidants such as vitamin C.

Further, recent studies published in *The Lancet* in August 1999, have shown that the levels of polyphenolics in chocolate can be as much as four times higher than those in tea. Given that these antioxidants in chocolate appear to be more effective than those in tea, then chocolate is one of the best sources of antioxidants in the diet.

Now some readers may be thinking, what about red wine, isn't that also high in these polyphenolic antioxidants we are talking about? Well, this is true, but wine also contains alcohol, which is a known carcinogen. A major review of the research studies on alcohol and breast cancer found that the risk of breast cancer was 40 to 70 percent higher in women who drank two or more glasses of alcoholic beverages per day. For this reason we believe any wine drinking should be limited to less than one glass a day—or better still, eat some chocolate instead.

Chocolate and Cholesterol, the "Bad" LDL and the "Good" HDL

These days we hear a lot about cholesterol. This is an important compound that the body needs to help build cell walls and manufacture many hormones, such as the sex hormones, and even vitamins. Cholesterol is made by the body and is also found in animal fats in the diet. Some dietary cholesterol is absorbed into the bloodstream as part of the digestion process. Before cholesterol can be transported through the bloodstream it must be combined with fats and proteins into particles called lipo-proteins. Low density lipo-proteins (or LDL) are known as the "bad" cholesterol. They are the artery blockers. The "good" or high density lipo-proteins (or HDL) are believed to scavenge the excess cholesterol from the bloodstream and carry it to the liver, where it is broken down.

One of the reasons it is not good to have high levels of LDL cholesterol in our blood is that when this cholesterol is oxidized by a free radical it cannot function properly. This leads to damage of the cells in the artery wall. As the body attempts to repair this damage, the artery is partly blocked. Thus oxidized LDL cholesterol promotes artery clogging. By having antioxidants in our diet we can prevent oxygen free radicals from damaging the LDL, thereby reducing its ability to damage artery walls and contributing to the build-up of plaque.

Laboratory experiments with the extracts from cocoa powder have shown that the polyphenols in cocoa strongly inhibit the oxidation of LDL. So, to maintain cardiovascular or heart health, it is not only important to maintain normal LDL cholesterol levels but also to maintain a normal rate of LDL cholesterol oxidation. One preliminary study found that the LDL cholesterol in blood taken from people *after* eating a small amount of nonfat cocoa was less likely to react with oxygen than LDL cholesterol taken from the same people *before* they ate nonfat cocoa. This finding was confirmed in subsequent study at the Pennsylvania State University. By testing the blood of 23 volunteers, scientists found that the antioxidant activity of the blood was increased after eating chocolate and that the time it took for the blood to oxidize was measurably longer. This clearly showed that eating chocolate could play a role in helping maintain cardiovascular health.

Chocolate's Polyphenolics and Heart Attack or Stroke

The polyphenolics in chocolate have been found to have another interesting effect. That is, they were found to decrease the blood platelet activation over a six-hour period after consuming a cocoa beverage. Platelets are the smallest of the red blood cells, but when activated can clump together and form clots to stop bleeding. It is thought that overactive platelets can increase the risk of blood clots causing heart attack or stroke. John quotes research from the University of California at Davis that suggests that flavonoid-rich foods may benefit the heart in this important way by damping the reactivity of the blood platelets. For this reason doctors have for some time now recommended that people at risk of heart attacks take a low dose of (baby) aspirin a day to reduce clotting. On the other hand, the aspirinlike effect of the polyphenolic compounds in cocoa can help decrease the risk of heart attack and stroke. In fact, regular intake of chocolate and cocoa products may contribute to an overall significantly lower risk of stroke.

John also found one study by nutritionist Carl L. Keen at the University of California, Davis, published in the July 2000 issue of *The American*

Journal of Clinical Nutrition, in which water, or cocoa (which was especially rich in procyanidins, the large molecule type polyphenols) or alcohol-free wine was given to groups of ten men and women. The researchers then sampled and tested the volunteers' blood two hours and six hours later. Although both the wine and the cocoa significantly delayed the blood-clotting time, only the cocoa protected the blood platelets from fragmentation.

In another study, Dr. Tissa Kappagoda at the School of Medicine at the University of California, Davis, found that procyanidins helped relax the inner surface of blood vessels. This relaxation effect can play a major part in cardiovascular health. In some people the relaxation mechanism is impaired. As a result they can have high blood pressure and atherosclerosis is exacerbated. In healthy blood vessels much of this relaxation is controlled by the production of a molecule known as nitric oxide. It now seems that certain compounds in chocolate actually increase the production of nitric oxide in the bloodstream, thereby relaxing the muscles lining blood vessels. It seems that the chocolate procyanidins can regulate enzyme activity that leads to an increase in the production of nitric oxide.

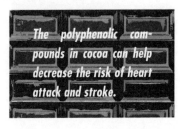

The polyphenolic compounds in cocoa can help decrease the risk of heart attack and stroke.

This mechanism has some similarities to the way the anti-impotence drug Viagra works, something perhaps the Aztecs knew about quite unwittingly all those years ago.

For most people, a moderate intake of chocolate over the long term may inhibit platelet activity, help prevent cholesterol oxidation and ultimately reduce the risk of heart and artery disease.

Anticancer Agents in Chocolate

But there is more to the polyphenol story for chocolate. Of the simpler flavonoids found in fermented cocoa beans, the one that occurs in the greatest concentration is a compound called epicatechin. This particular flavonoid has been found to have anticancer activity. In fact, in test animals, epicatechin has been found to protect against gamma radiation, a type of ionizing radiation which causes damage to chromosomes. Epicate-

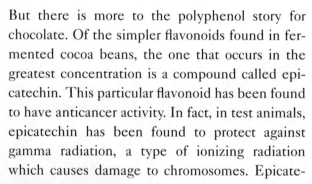

chin also prevented the ability of certain components of tobacco smoke to interact with DNA, and other studies have shown that this powerful flavonoid can inhibit chemically in-

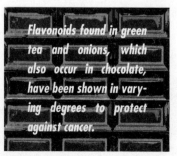

Flavonoids found in green tea and onions, which also occur in chocolate, have been shown in varying degrees to protect against cancer.

duced skin cancers in test animals such as mice.

While epicatechin is the most common of the flavonoids in cocoa, others have also been studied. Flavonoids found in green tea and onions, which also occur in chocolate, have been shown in varying degrees to protect against cancer. Cocoa also contains another anticancer agent called ferulic acid. Ferulic acid is used topically in skin lotions and sunscreens and has been found to reduce the side effects of chemotherapy treatment for cancer. To us, the evidence is becoming clearer that chocolate is one of nature's special anticancer foods. When it comes to a choice between chocolate and red wine, in health terms, we believe chocolate wins every time.

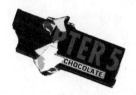

But Isn't Chocolate Fattening?

Chocolate and the Guilt Factor

When you think of chocolates, what comes to mind? A special memory of a romantic evening? The wonderful expression of joy and happiness on your mother's face, perhaps when she opened the box of chocolates on Mother's Day? (Chocolate was a standard Mother's Day gift in our house!) And of course, isn't a heart-shaped box of chocolates often the gift of choice for that very special friend on Valentine's Day? If, on the other hand, someone brings a tray of chocolates for morning tea at work, or when a plate of chocolates is brought in for afternoon tea at a social gathering, or after a meal, you may tend to think in terms of, "Oh no! This is fattening! I like it but, NO!"

For many women (and until recently I was one of them) our conscience tells us that eating chocolate will make us put on weight, and what will our coworkers think? Don't you take any pride in your appearance? But just as you let your conscience slide into oblivion and you are about to succumb to one of the few legal pleasures left, a voice beside you whispers something like "I hope you'll be able to walk out the door this afternoon" and snickering soon echoes around the room. Or, if you are the kind-hearted soul trying to bring some happiness into people's lives, you may be told (jokingly, of course!), "What are you trying to do? Make us all fat?"

One of my favorite experiences is one that it seems only women can share. It's when a group of women secretly congregate to a known spot and say among the sighs of those in chocolate heaven, "I know I shouldn't be doing this, but..." and her friends give sympathetic nods of agreement as they indulge in the sweet creaminess of the sacred chocolate platter. (Most men never understand this, as they seem to have no in-built chocolate-guilt factor!) Why this need for secrecy and guilt? Is chocolate a food that will make someone fat and help them put on weight? Why do we give it as a present for a special occasion? Have we created a situation for the receivers of our beautiful chocolate boxes to feel guilty at a time when they should be joyful?

We all know that chocolate is a pleasurable food to eat. No matter what your body shape or size, very few people can resist the call of sweet, creamy, milky chocolate. I am no exception, and so it came as no surprise to find that one day I found myself casually browsing through the chocolate aisle of the local supermarket, indulging in day-dreams of kingdoms built entirely out of choco-late. It was a rather hot day and I was wearing clothes that revealed a little more than usual. An older, male voice soon startled me out of my fan-tasies. "Hey, love," it said, "you don't want to be looking at those . . . they'll make you fat!" I swung around and stared at the short, squat middle-aged man who was speaking to me. His potbelly and double chins might have been proof of chocolate's effect on him, but then chips, beer, and a much too sedentary lifestyle in front of the TV might also have caused them. I stumbled out that I was actu-ally looking for carob—isn't that a healthier alter-native?—and walked away as fast as I could.

Here we see that chocolate occupies a rather

ambiguous position in the world of food. It is the best of foods and the worst of foods; it has connotations both of reward and luxury, as well as HIGH FAT, unhealthy, a forbidden fruit. We have in chocolate both the treat and the temptation. Naughty, but nice. Maybe Eve was tempted with a cocoa bean, not an apple! So, how should we regard chocolate? Is it just a food for a special occasion, or to be enjoyed as an occasional luxury? Should we use chocolate as a snack that can boost energy levels? (We often don't feel as bad about having an extra cup of coffee to keep us awake as we do about having a few nibbles of chocolate.) Or is our yearning for chocolate a desire for an unhealthy fattening food that we need to avoid?

The Fat Myth Exposed

Well, there's no doubt that many of us have the perception that chocolate will put on weight. But let's have a look at the situation more closely. John found a study published in 1994 in the prestigious *American Journal of Clinical Nutrition*, pointing out that, on average, chocolate contributes only 0.7 to 1.4 percent of our total daily energy intake. So, just on this figure alone, we can

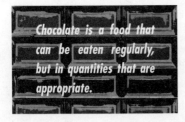

Chocolate is a food that can be eaten regularly, but in quantities that are appropriate.

see that for the average person chocolate consumption is not likely to be the cause of an overweight body shape. Of course, there may be some of us who do eat quite a lot of chocolate, and chocolate is an energy-dense food. That simply means that if we eat a lot of chocolate, and we don't exercise a lot or burn up that energy, then ultimately we will gain weight. But does this mean that chocolate is fattening? Well, no! Not really. What it means is that chocolate is meant to be eaten in a certain portion size. It's a food that can be eaten regularly, but in quantities that are appropriate. I don't know of anybody who would like to eat a whole block of butter in one sitting, but butter spread on a piece of fresh bread is delightful. It's the same principle with chocolate. Eat a family-size block in one sitting, do no exercise, and you'll probably feel slightly queasy and put on a little weight. Do this every day and you'll put on quite a lot of weight!

Chocolate vs. Other Snacks

Let us consider, for example, a typical 50 g (around 2 oz) chocolate bar. This would contain more antioxidants than a glass of red wine, but it would also contribute to the diet about 1100 kJ or 260 kilocalories to our energy intake. This is approximately 10 to 15 percent of the daily calorie needs for the average person. However, such a chocolate bar may contain four segments that could be eaten as a sweet snack at four different times during the day, and each segment would contain fewer calories than the average small sweet biscuit or cookie. If we ate the whole 50 g (2 oz) block of chocolate in one sitting, we would probably feel quite satiated, and we would not feel hungry for some time afterwards. On the other hand, if we ate four small sweet biscuits or cookies, we may still feel like eating more a short time later. This illustrates the subtle difference between eating something like chocolate and eating a food which delivers the same amount of calories but mainly from carbohydrates.

74

We will find out in the next chapter that many carbohydrate foods stimulate insulin production and excess insulin circulating in the blood can increase our desire for more food. Eating a high carbohydrate snack may leave us with a craving to eat even more—and what happens? We find that we haven't just eaten one cookie, but we have eaten two or three of them! We believe it is this subtle difference that has surprised many people when they've changed to eating chocolate at the end of a meal and found that they had maintained or lost weight. This is because they are now not eating high-calorie pastries and desserts after the meal.

Chocolate contains the same amount of calories per gram as most sweet cookies, potato chips or corn chips, and fewer calories per gram than most nuts. But most of us would not experience the same guilt after eating 50 g (2 oz) of potato chips as we would after eating the same amount of chocolate. When you think about it, it is quite easy to eat 100 g (about 4 oz) of salted peanuts or 100 g (4 oz) of cookies during the course of the day. In these cases we would be consuming twice as many calories as we would if we ate our entire 50 g (2 oz) chocolate bar.

When we think of desserts—what foods come to mind: an apple crumble, vanilla slice, cheesecake, blueberry muffin, a fruit pie, a Danish, a cake, or maybe an iced doughnut? A typical serving of all these desserts contains roughly the same amount of calories as our 50 g (2 oz) chocolate bar. And 50 g (2 oz) of chocolate is the *maximum* amount of chocolate that we recommend per day. Some days we would have half that amount, i.e., 25 g (1 oz), and sometimes we'd have only two or three small pieces of chocolate after dinner,

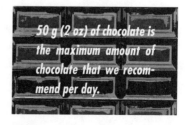

50 g (2 oz) of chocolate is the maximum amount of chocolate that we recommend per day.

amounting to a mere 10 or 12 g (½ oz) of chocolate for the day, as a satisfying replacement for dessert.

Eating just one dessert a day, especially if we have a scoop of ice-cream or cream with it, will usually contribute more calories than our chocolate ration. And when we have more than one serving, or an extra large serving, or eat dessert at more than one meal, that is when we can put on the calories. Even a single custard tart contributes 30 percent more calories than 50 g (2 oz) of chocolate, with a single lamington supplying about 75 percent of the calories or the same as about 35 g (1¼ oz) of milk chocolate or 40 g (1½ oz) of dark chocolate. So we feel we are much better off, weight and nutrition wise, eating a small amount of chocolate a day instead of dessert, and having desserts, including rich chocolate desserts, only at special occasions or as an extra special treat.

Different Fats Have Different Properties

Now you might be saying to yourself—but isn't the fat in chocolate saturated fat? Would I not be better off in terms of my cholesterol levels eating a low-fat carbohydrate dessert? Well, that very question was checked out by Dr. Penny Kris-Etherton and coworkers in the Department of Nutrition at Pennsylvania State University. They fed 42 healthy young men with normal cholesterol levels a controlled diet for three weeks, which included either a 46 g (about 1¾ oz) milk chocolate bar or a high carbohydrate snack of the same energy, and measured their cholesterol before and after the diet. Compared to when they were eating the low-fat carbohydrate snack, the chocolate eaters had improved cholesterol and blood lipid profiles with lower triglyceride levels and higher "good" HDL cholesterol levels. There was no adverse effect on the "bad" LDL cholesterol despite the increase in total fat and saturated fat in the diet.

The fat in chocolate comes from cocoa butter which, since it comes from a plant, naturally contains no cholesterol. Cocoa butter consists mainly of three types of dietary fatty acids: palmitic and stearic, which are saturated fats, and oleic acid, which is a monounsaturated fat just like the type found in olive oil. Each of these types of fats make up approximately one-third of the total fat. So we can see, one-third of the fat in chocolate is of the oleic acid (or olive oil) type. Another third is stearic acid; although this is a saturated fat, it does not raise plasma cholesterol levels. It has now been discovered that stearic acid is converted to monounsaturated oleic acid via a special enzyme in the liver. The fat is then recirculated in a form that does not raise our cholesterol.

Some dark chocolates contain milk fat (butter oil) and of course in milk chocolate there is also fat from the milk, and we know that these sorts of fats (milk fats) do tend to raise cholesterol levels. However, in several studies now, where subjects were fed milk chocolate in very high amounts, the level of LDL cholesterol, the kind of cholesterol that has been linked to heart disease, did not increase in those people on that particular diet. So we can see that the good fats in chocolate seem to neutralize the small amount of the bad fats from the milk fat.

The third fat, palmitic acid, is a typical saturated fat. However, in nature we find that most natural foods contain a mixture of fats with some saturated fats and it seems that saturated fats are important in the diet. For example, saturated fats seem to protect us from skin cancer. Studies at Sydney University have shown that when test animals such as mice were fed saturated fat in the diet, in this case from butter, it was very difficult to induce skin cancers using ultraviolet light. However, when the diet of the test animals was changed over to polyunsaturated fats, the skin cancers grew like mushrooms. On reflection, as the cocoa

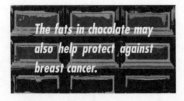
The fats in chocolate may also help protect against breast cancer.

beans grow in the hot tropics we can see that nature has again provided a perfectly balanced food for those sorts of conditions.

The fats in chocolate may also help protect against breast cancer. As we've noted, two-thirds of the fat in chocolate is effectively oleic acid, as found in olive oil. It has been known for some time now that in countries where olive oil consumption is high, breast cancer rates are much lower. By the same token, in countries where polyunsaturated fats are consumed, some researchers have observed higher rates of breast cancer. This observation has been borne out in animal studies of breast cancer. Increased mammary tumors have been observed primarily when animals have been fed high amounts of polyunsaturated fats of the omega-6 type which occur in high levels in sunflower oil, safflower oil, and soy bean oil.

The Drawbacks of Some Vegetable Oils

Chocolates compose about 14–18 percent of snack foods eaten, the bulk being savory snacks such as potato chips or corn chips, cookies, and pastry type foods. Most of these foods are made with vegetable oils. To survive the heating processes and to make them more like harder, saturated fats (such as butter and animal fats, which were traditionally used in making these foods), some vegetable oils are now partially altered by a process using hydrogen gas to form trans-fatty acids. These new hydrogenated fatty acids are quite different from the fats that occur naturally.

Researchers are now linking the consumption of these fats with diseases such as cancer and heart disease. This has prompted some high profile nutritionists to call for the labeling of the trans-fatty acids content of foods high in these types of fats. John refers to a study of the trans-fatty acid content of foods in 1983 by Dr. Mary Enig from the University of Maryland which found that of 25 samples of cookies or biscuits analyzed, a quarter contained more than 30 percent trans-fatty acids in the fat. In pastries the trans-fatty acid levels ranged up to 32 percent of the fat, while in French fries up to 35 percent of the fat was trans-fatty acids. When we take these facts into consideration, chocolate probably shapes up pretty well as an alternative healthier snack food.

One of the surprises of Dr. Enig's study was that out of the 220 foods analyzed in her survey, the highest level of trans-fatty acids of 38.6 percent was found in the fat of a carob malt ball. This highlights an unfortunate misconception regarding chocolate. Because of chocolate's poor health image, particularly concerns over its caffeine content, many health-conscious people have chosen to eat carob-based confectionery or snacks. Carob comes from the pods of the carob tree, which is a type of locust bean. It has a flavor very similar to chocolate and also contains polyphenolic type antioxidants, as does chocolate. However, it does not have the same cocoa fat which gives the wonderful mouth-feel of chocolate. So when carob confectionery is made, hydrogenated vegetable fats are usually used. Unfortunately many of us, who have been thinking we were eating a healthy confectionery, in actual fact have probably been eating a food that was far worse for our hearts and general health than chocolate.

Choose Your Chocolate Carefully

Similar high levels of trans-fatty acids or artificially made short-chain fatty acids are likely to be found in any of the compound chocolate confectionery, and in the cheaper chocolates made using hydrogenated vegetable fats as a substitute for cocoa butter. While these foods may contain the beneficial polyphenolics and minerals of chocolate, we feel that the trans-fatty acids and atherogenic short-chain fats that are found in the hydrogenated vegetable oils used to compose them are best avoided. These cheaper types of chocolate made with cocoa butter substitutes are far less desirable from a health perspective. In Europe, some chocolate manufacturers blend hydrogenated vegetable fats in with the cocoa butter, so read the labels carefully. If the ingredients list includes "vegetable oils" the chocolate is best left on the shelf, in our view.

Compound type chocolates are commonly used to coat muesli bars, and nuts and fruits, in the cheaper lines. The equipment required to coat these items is much simpler for the manufacturer when compound chocolate is used, because the melting point of hydrogenated fat mixtures is relatively

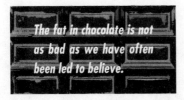

The fat in chocolate is not as bad as we have often been led to believe.

easy to control. On the other hand, the melting point of proper chocolate fat is such that special tempering equipment is required in the process to give the chocolate its characteristic melt-in-the-mouth feel.

It is highly likely that we will be hearing a lot more about trans fats in the future. In researching this book, John found that in 1999 researchers from the prestigious Harvard School of Public Health in Boston reported that on a gram for gram basis the adverse effects of trans fats appears to be much stronger than that of saturated fat—they were found to be almost twice as harmful. They found that 63 to 75 percent of the trans fats in the diet of Americans came from baked goods, fried fast foods, and other prepared foods, with the balance coming from margarines. The researchers point out that the consumption of one doughnut at breakfast (3.2 g [⅛ oz] of trans fats) and one large order of French fries at lunch (6.8 g [¼ oz] of trans fats) adds 10 g (⅓ oz) of pure trans fats to the diet.

John found another study, published in the *New England Journal of Medicine* in 1999, in which Dr. Alice Lichtenstein and coworkers from the Jean Meyer U.S. Department of Agriculture Human Nutrition Research Center on Aging at Tufts University in Boston found that trans fats in hydrogenated vegetable oils cause the body to produce a particularly atherogenic type of cholesterol known as lipoprotein "a," written Lp(a). High levels of this lipoprotein are strongly associated with an increased risk of developing heart and artery disease. On the other hand, saturated fats in the diet were found to lower the Lp(a) levels in the blood. These findings support the view that a balance of fats, including saturated fats, are beneficial and that these fats are best obtained from natural sources with the minimum of processing.

Chocolate Shapes Up Well

When all is said and done, in our view, the fat in chocolate is not as bad as we have often been led to believe. Sure, chocolate is about 30 percent fat, the same as cheddar cheese, and 50 g (2 oz) of chocolate would provide about 15 g (½ oz) of fat in our diet. Putting this in perspective, this is the same amount of fat as in a single serving of butter or margarine (one tablespoon) that we would spread on our bread. And how many servings of these fats would we have in a day? When we look for other sources of fat in our diet, according to the United States 1987–1998 National Food Consumption Survey, 30 percent of our dietary fats comes from meats, 22 percent from grains (in biscuits, crackers, cookies, cakes, and pies), and 20 percent from milk and dairy products. We feel that these foods, together with fried foods, butter and margarine, are the foods we need to cut back on in terms of reducing our fat intake and weight control. Chocolate intake accounted for only about 1 percent of the fat in the American diet (and most other Western-style diets, too), and as we have shown, the fat in chocolate is more akin to the healthy fat found in olive oil. When you think about it, a chocolate a day (instead of dessert) may not only keep the bathroom scales at bay but also the heart doctor away.

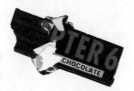

Chocolate Is No Ordinary Sweet

The image of a young woman with very long legs and a perfectly flat stomach suddenly appears on the TV screen. The conversation around the dinner table quiets as people strain to hear what this vision of loveliness has to say. It turns out that this is an advertisement for an artificial sweetener and, of course, the woman maintains her perfect hourglass shape by using this particular brand of artificial sweetener. No added calories, no worries, is the message portrayed throughout the ad. This ad and many others like it were typical when artificial sweeteners were being promoted in the popular media.

Sugar vs. Artificial Sweeteners

There has been much debate over the years about the health benefits (or nonbenefits) of including sugar products in our diet. Growing up in tropical northern Australia, being surrounded by lush green fields of sugarcane and hearing the cane trains go by at night, I took sugar for granted as a natural part of life. In fact, the theme "sugar—it's a natural part of life" was taken on by the sugar industry as a campaign against the artificial sweetener manufacturers a few years ago. Since the rise of these artificial sweeteners there has been much talk about the ugly side effects of both products— sugar and its imitators. People are obviously concerned about their health as far as sugar is concerned. Chocolate manufacturers have caught hold of this trend and there are now chocolate bars available with artificial sweetening. Most chocolate, however, is still made with natural sugar and it is this type of chocolate that we are looking at. This chapter will give you insights into the biological workings of sugar and carbohydrate in the diet, and how this affects our health. As always, the theme of this book is chocolate as a health food—as long as it's eaten in moderation!

When we talk about chocolate being healthy, perhaps one of the first questions people ask is,

"But what about all that sugar?" And it's true—many chocolates can contain 50 percent or more of sugar. For this reason chocolate has not been recommended for people with diabetes. However, recent research is now changing this perspective on chocolate. Sugar, sometimes called sucrose, is a natural carbohydrate that is found in sugarcane and many other natural foods (such as peanuts, which contain about 6 percent sucrose). What scientists are now realizing is that it's not so much the amount of sugar that we eat but the amount of total carbohydrate that we eat, and how this carbohydrate is converted to glucose in the body, which can cause the excess body fat problem. Fat is a word that now has a very negative connotation to many people. Women especially can be almost phobic about the amount of fat they let into their diet.

What we need to realize is that fat doesn't only come in one form. Many people today follow diets that talk about less fat and more carbohydrate. Here we explain how excess sugar, or excess carbohydrate, is converted into fat.

How Excess Sugar Converts into Fat

Glucose is the fuel that our body runs on. Whether we eat pure sugar, such as in a candy or a soft drink, or we eat a piece of fruit or piece of bread or some pasta, all these foods are converted during the digestion process into glucose, which is absorbed into the bloodstream. Have you ever noticed that when you eat a piece of bread, if you keep chewing for a while, the bread actually loses some of its salty taste and begins to taste sweet? This is because the complex carbohydrates in the bread are being broken down by enzymes into glucose. As a result, after we eat a carbohydrate food there is a surge of glucose levels in the blood. How large this surge is for a standard portion of carbohydrate is called the glycemic index (G.I.). If the G.I. of the food is low, i.e. less than around 50 units, the food is releasing glucose only slowly into the bloodstream at a rate that can be utilized by cells in the body for energy. *When we eat these low G.I. types of foods, one of the reasons it is harder to put on weight is because our bodies are using up this energy, rather than storing it as excess fat.*

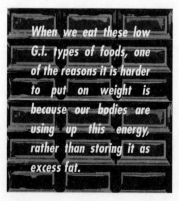

When we eat these low G.I. types of foods, one of the reasons it is harder to put on weight is because our bodies are using up this energy, rather than storing it as excess fat.

Most people have heard of insulin, and know that it is related to diabetes. It is found in the bloodstream, and its main purpose is to promote the entry of glucose into cells. Some insulin is also used to convert glucose to glycogen in our muscles, where it is stored as the fuel for our daily activities. When our glycogen stores are full, insulin converts any excess glucose into fat, which is stored in fat cells throughout the body. If a food has a high glycemic index, say above 70 G.I. units, it means that when it is digested it releases a large surge of glucose into the bloodstream. Foods such as French fries and baked potatoes, doughnuts, waffles, certain types of rice and bread, and refined breakfast cereals such as cornflakes and rice puffs, all have high G.I. values. They release their energy quickly into the body as glucose. This extra high level of blood sugar stimulates the pancreas to release more insulin into the bloodstream to bring the blood glucose level down. The reason for this is that excess glucose is actually dangerous for us. If left in the blood it can cause damage to the eyes, kidneys, nerves, and liver. Indeed, these are the symptoms, or effects, of diabetes, which is a disease where the body is producing insufficient insulin to convert the glucose in the blood. This results in high blood sugar levels.

The problem when we eat high G.I. foods is

that unless we have been engaging in vigorous physical exercise and have depleted our glycogen stores in our muscles, then this glucose will be converted into fat. Not only that, this surge of insulin can leave higher levels than normal of insulin circulating in the blood; which in turn produces the effect of making us feel hungry again, only a short time later. This in turn means that we are more than likely going to eat more food and thereby put on more weight. On the other hand, low G.I. foods tend to be more satisfying and do not promote the same level of hormonal and metabolic changes that encourage excessive food intake. As a result we have a tendency to eat less and therefore control our weight.

Weight control seems to be an issue that concerns women more than men. Most women have dieted at least once in their lives. There are even weight control diets tailored specifically for special occasions, like the bride's two-weeks-before-the-wedding diet. I'm sure many women have half starved themselves before an important social occasion, just so they can squeeze into that chic little dress! I haven't, however, seen too many diets for men. You also don't usually see scales in men's bathrooms, or a height–weight chart in a men's public toilet (I asked my husband about this). However, while weight control may be deemed a totally feminine area, men also should be concerned about their weight health.

In one study conducted at the Children's Hospital, Boston, and published recently in the journal *Pediatrics*, overweight teenage boys were given a specially formulated low G.I. breakfast. After that, they were allowed to eat whatever they liked throughout the day. At the end of the investigation it was found that the teenagers had actually lost weight over the period of the study. Furthermore, it now appears that eating a lot of high G.I. foods over a period of time can not only make us fat but also increase our risk of heart disease. It has also been discovered that too many high G.I. foods in our diet can cause our body to produce insufficient "good" HDL types of cholesterol to balance the "bad" LDL cholesterol which can clog up our arteries. These are good reasons to cut back on the high G.I. foods and add more low G.I. foods to our diet.

High G.I. Foods and Diabetes

High G.I. carbohydrate foods are also linked to the development of type 2 diabetes. When we eat a lot of these foods regularly in our diet, the resulting continued production of high levels of insulin by the pancreas seems to result in cells becoming resistant to insulin. This means that more insulin than usual has to be produced to get the excess glucose out of the blood. This in turn overloads the pancreas to the point where it becomes exhausted and now unable to produce sufficient insulin to convert the glucose from the food we have eaten. We now have the situation of type 2 diabetes.

While not everyone with insulin resistance will go on to develop diabetes, high levels of insulin in the blood stimulates the liver to produce higher levels of the "bad" LDL cholesterol which tends to clog up our arteries. In fact, the American Heart Association research found that high levels of insulin in the blood was the most statistically significant predictor of heart attack risk—equal to or more significant than cholesterol levels.

What Do We Need to Do?

To combat these debilitating diseases we need to include low G.I. foods such as pasta and spaghetti, whole grain breads, legumes, peanuts, and raw apples and pears, in our diets. We also need to eat fewer high G.I. carbohydrate foods. This is one of the best ways of avoiding high insulin levels. Glycemic index is a way of classifying mainly carbohydrate foods such as candy, pastries, cookies, breads, and breakfast cereals. It is not as relevant to high protein foods such as meat, fish, and dairy products, which usually have very low G.I. values. Fruits and vegetables can have varying G.I. values from low to high, but eating a variety of these health-giving foods with our meals will automatically balance out the G.I. effect.

The $64,000 Question

So now for the $64,000 question. Where does chocolate fit in this picture? It may surprise you to find that milk chocolate has a relatively low G.I. In fact, the average value for milk chocolate was 45 G.I. units, with a plain chocolate reported as having a G.I. of 49 units. This means that these chocolate products would be classified in the low G.I. food range; that is, foods with G.I. values

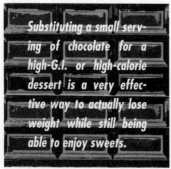

of less than 50 units. The important point that comes from this is that while chocolate is relatively high in sugar, it actually has a lower G.I. than sugar by itself (G.I. 66 units) and can be used as a pleasurable treat, even by most people with diabetes. We need to remember of course that chocolate products are usually very energy dense foods; that is, they contain a large amount of energy per gram. Therefore, we don't need to eat very much of them—remember the theme of this book! However, they can play a small but nonetheless pleasurable and guilt-free part in our diet. In fact, substituting a small serving of chocolate for a high-G.I. or high-calorie dessert is a very effective way to actually lose weight while still being able to enjoy sweets. When we consider the relatively high-G.I. effects of many of the desserts that we like, such as cakes, cookies, and candy containing glucose (check the ingredients list, as glucose has a very high G.I. of 100 units), we would be helping to lower the overall glycemic index of our meal if we chose to eat a small piece or two of chocolate instead of these foods.

We need to remember of course that most chocolates

Substituting a small serving of chocolate for a high-G.I. or high-calorie dessert is a very effective way to actually lose weight while still being able to enjoy sweets.

with a soft, sweet filling will have a higher G.I. than plain chocolate. For example, a chocolate-covered caramel and nougat bar may have a G.I. of around 62 units. Chocolates with sweet fillings containing glucose or glucose syrups (a cheap sugar substitute) will have an even higher G.I., and we recommend that these chocolates only be eaten occasionally as special treats. These are the types of chocolates usually found in beautifully packaged boxes, and are a great way to enhance romance on an anniversary or other special occasion.

The Importance of Chromium

There is yet another aspect to the sweet side of chocolate. John reports that scientists have found that for the proper metabolism of glucose, the body requires trace amounts of the mineral chromium. Dr. Milton Crane, Emeritus Professor of Medicine at the Loma Linda University, points out that every time we eat candy made with refined sugar or foods made with white flour or white rice, we lose more chromium than we take in and gradually over time we deplete the body's stores of chromium. Scientists at the United States Department of Agricul-

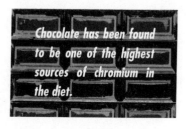

Chocolate has been found to be one of the highest sources of chromium in the diet.

ture's Human Nutrition Research Center found that when test animals were given a chromium-deficient diet they had much higher serum insulin levels. The researchers also found in an earlier study with humans that when individuals with type 2 diabetes were given chromium supplements in their diets it had a significant beneficial effect, reducing both their blood glucose and insulin levels. The leader of these studies, Dr. Richard Anderson, points out chromium is a nutrient notably lacking in our diets.

Chocolate has been found to be one of the highest sources of chromium in the diet. In a recent survey of chromium levels in 150 common foods, dark chocolate was found to have the second highest level of chromium of all the foods analyzed, a level ten times higher than whole wheat. (The highest level of chromium was found in a yeast spread.) The chocolate-based beverage analyzed also had a very high level of chromium compared with most other foods. On the other hand, foods such as sugar and white flour had no detectable chromium in them.

Does Chocolate Cause Tooth Decay?

Sweets and refined foods are also associated with tooth decay, as our dentist will remind us. However, chocolate is no ordinary sweet. The human and animal studies that have been carried out to measure how much tooth decay different foods cause have shown that chocolate has only a very mild potential to cause tooth decay, about the same as whole-meal bread and bran cereal. When we eat foods containing sugars or other carbohydrates and do not clean our teeth straightaway, bacteria in our mouth ferment food particles around our teeth to acids. Dr. Martin Curzon from a university department of Pediatric Dentistry in the U.K., writing in *Chocolate and Cocoa: Health and Nutrition*, points out that the cocoa in chocolate contains natural chemicals that inhibit the bacteria that release the acids that attack our teeth. Other factors in cocoa actually make the enamel on our teeth more resistant to acid attack. Since milk also contains factors that inhibit tooth decay, it is not surprising that milk chocolate is about 30 percent less cariogenic (decay causing) than dark chocolate. The tooth enamel dissolving power of

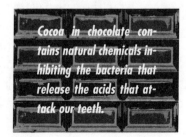

Cocoa in chocolate contains natural chemicals inhibiting the bacteria that release the acids that attack our teeth.

milk chocolate was found to be less than that of whole-meal bread and only about one-quarter of the dissolving power of white bread or cornflakes. When milk chocolate was ranked against snack foods in animal studies it had a lower cariogenic index than bread, cakes, French fries, bananas, and even raisins. If eaten in moderation, chocolate should not be considered as a worrying cause of tooth decay.

Chocolate and Acne?—A Myth Debunked

Another thing we can worry about with chocolate is acne. It is a widely held belief that eating chocolate will cause pimples to erupt or make acne worse. Yet it may come as a surprise that there seems to *not* be a lot of scientific evidence to support this. In one study conducted over six years at the Missouri University Health Services, student patients with acne were questioned about the foods that they thought caused their acne. Those who thought that chocolate, nuts, or cola were the cause were provided with and consumed large quantities of these foods under supervision. The author of the study concluded "to the constant amazement of both the patients and medical students, absolutely no major flares of acne were produced by the foods." Other studies have found similar results. The American Dietetic Association, in its 1996 consumer publication *Complete Food and Nutrition Guide*, described the view that chocolate causes acne as a myth: "That misconception has captured the attention of teens for years. However, hormonal changes during adolescence are the usual causes of acne, not chocolate."

Nutritionists and dieticians have always been concerned about people eating too many sweets, and traditionally chocolate has been placed in the same basket. But chocolate is no ordinary sweet, high in empty calories. Instead, chocolate is an amazingly functional sweet, providing important nutrients as well as pleasure. So enjoy!

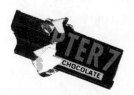

The Chocolate Lifestyle

A remote tropical island with white sandy beaches and tantalizingly clear waters seizes your attention as you flip through the latest magazine. "Is this the lifestyle for you?" asks the promoter of the resort featured in the advertisement. Lifestyle, it's a word that seems to have crept into our language and everyday use. Advertisers promote things from furniture to health retreats to improve our lifestyle, while medical authorities recommend we have a healthy diet and get plenty of exercise. Are there good reasons to change some of the sedentary habits that we love so well, like sitting in front of the TV for two hours after work, unwinding? What are the benefits of a healthy lifestyle, we may ask ourselves? Well, long life is alleged to be one of them, but maybe this is not an important focus for us at the moment. Well, what about a better sex life, more energy, well-toned muscles, less cellulite? The last thing you'd expect to find associated with these health attributes is *chocolate*. Yet chocolate can actually help us to have a better lifestyle.

Chocolate epitomizes a food that gives both enjoyment and health. It is also a food that must be enjoyed for what it is, and not used in excess. More is not better. In this regard chocolate can be symbolic of a "balanced" lifestyle that promotes health and quality of life. We've already suggested that finishing a meal with a piece or two of chocolate can totally replace the need for fattening desserts such as rich puddings, tarts, cheesecake, iced doughnuts, and other high-calorie sweets. So what else should we be eating for our meals to make up a really healthy diet? This chapter explores some of the vast array of health-giving foods that, together with other lifestyle factors, such as enjoyable exercise and rest, can lay the foundation for a long and energy-filled life.

Green Leafy Vegetables — Choose Them First

Perhaps one of the most profound revelations of the latest nutrition research is the far-reaching health benefits of green leafy vegetables. As John points out, leading nutrition researchers, such as Professor David Jenkins at the Faculty of Medicine at the University of Toronto, are now discovering that green leafy vegetables should be a major part of our diet. In fact, we should have three or four, or perhaps more, servings of green leafy vegetables each day. Now, you might be thinking, I can't possibly eat four servings of lettuce or salad a day. As with any diet, the secret of success is variety. Not only can we have our greens in the form of salads, but we can have them steamed and as stir fries. A whole cabbage or cos lettuce can be chopped up, placed in a pan with some olive oil, and simmered gently for a few minutes. Simmering and steaming will greatly reduce the bulk of the green leafy vegetables.

The addition of olive oil to stir fries makes many of the important antioxidant vitamins more readily available in the body. Broccoli, cabbage, spinach, bok

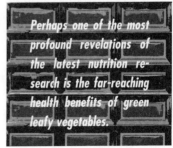

Perhaps one of the most profound revelations of the latest nutrition research is the far-reaching health benefits of green leafy vegetables.

choy, silver beet, chard, watercress, wombok, cos lettuce, and even ordinary iceberg lettuce can be eaten this way. We can also try some of the other Mediterranean greens such as kale, endive, and rocket, a green leafy vegetable with a very pleasant nutty taste.

Greens are very good sources of not only antioxidants but also minerals such as calcium, magnesium, and potassium. We noted earlier that many researchers believe that one possible cause of chocolate craving is a deficiency in magnesium. By ensuring that we have plenty of greens each day, our body will have an ample supply of magnesium. This will reduce the craving for chocolate and enable us to enjoy chocolate for what it is.

The Importance of Vegetables and Fruit in Our Diet

Vegetables should be a major part of our diet; particularly brightly colored vegetables such as green beans, asparagus, celery, peas, capsicum, brussels sprouts, leeks, zucchini and cauliflower, and the red-yellow vegetables such as beetroot, sweet potato, pumpkin and carrot and sweet corn. We should also include liberal servings of fresh salad vegetables such as cucumber, radish, and tomato. Tomatoes are one of the best sources of a powerful antioxidant called lycopene which is believed to help protect against prostate cancer. Remember to also include liberal amounts of tomatoes in your stir fries as cooking the tomato increases the lycopene benefit. Flavor vegetables such as onion and garlic are also important. It is believed that four grams of garlic a day (about one clove) can help the body protect against cancer and also help us to keep our blood pressure in the normal range.

Whenever you are tempted to eat a snack, or need a light meal, think of fruit. Fruits come in a mouth-watering array of flavors including, believe it or not, chocolate, the flavor of chocolate pudding fruit (black sapote). We are probably familiar with the common fruits such as apples, pears, apricots, oranges, plums, grapes, melons, bananas, etc. However, there are many other fruits we should try to include in our diet, from purple mangosteen (described as the Queen of Tropical Fruits), to blueberries and billberries which are rich in antioxidants and can help slow down the deterioration of our eyesight with age. The delicious lychee is high in vitamin C, while pawpaws and mangos are high in both vitamin C and vitamin A. Strawberries and kiwifruit are other good sources of vitamin C, while blackberries are good sources of both calcium and magnesium.

Cereals—And Choose the Right Ones

Another important part of our diet should be whole-grain cereals, particularly pasta and rice. Whole-grain cereals are another good source of magnesium because the magnesium tends to be concentrated in the bran parts of the cereal which is otherwise discarded during the modern milling and refining processes. By using whole-grain cereal products we are getting good sources of vitamins, minerals, and fiber.

One of the best cereals to eat is buckwheat. It is an excellent source of the flavonoid rutin, which can help keep our cholesterol levels down and normalize blood pressure. It may also help protect the body against cancer.

Some breakfast cereals such as cornflakes and rice puffs (which are refined carbohydrates) have a very high G.I. and are best used only occasionally. Modern commercial breads are another food that is perhaps best eaten in moderation, as again they have a relatively high G.I. compared to their old-fashioned whole-grain counterparts that were eaten by our grandparents. On the other hand, brown- and long-grain rice, and the var-

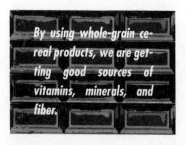

By using whole-grain cereal products, we are getting good sources of vitamins, minerals, and fiber.

ious pastas and spaghettis, are good low G.I. cereal foods to include in our diet.

Legumes, Too

Another food group that should be part of our daily diet is the legumes. These are the beans and peas such as butter beans, adzuki beans, lima beans, black-eyed beans, kidney beans, cannellini beans, borlotti beans, broad beans, mung beans, soy beans, lentils, and chickpeas. Dr. David Jenkins, who is Professor of Nutritional Sciences and Medicine at the University of Toronto in Canada, and who first discovered the importance of the glycemic index, points out that on the Japanese island of Okinawa, the diet is high in green leafy vegetables and soya beans. This is significant because this island has the highest percentage of people, anywhere in the world, living over one hundred years.

Legumes, and in particular soya beans, which have been studied the most, are found to have very effective cholesterol-lowering properties and appear to offer substantial protection against heart disease. One of the reasons for this is that soy is a particularly rich source of natural compounds called isoflavones, which not only lower cholesterol, but are strong antioxidants which can help maintain bone health and protect against cancer. Soya beans have to be cooked very thoroughly but it is possible to buy soy-based products such as tempeh and tofu which are good protein foods for savories and stir fries. Chickpeas, also known as garbanzos or Bengal gram, have similar health benefits to soy, but are easier to prepare. Hommos (or hummus) is a tasty purée made from cooked chickpeas. Roasted chickpeas are also sold in some shops.

Nuts, Just a Few

Nuts are another food that we should include as part of our daily menu. Like chocolate, nuts are high in fat, so we don't need to eat a lot of them. In his reading, John found that many studies, such as a 1998 Harvard Medical School study of 22,000 men, are finding that nuts such as walnuts, macadamia nuts, pecans, and almonds, and even the common peanut, which is also an excellent source of magnesium, offer a significant degree of protection against heart disease. It has also been suggested that we eat a couple of brazil nuts every day as a natural source of selenium, another important antioxidant that our body needs to protect against heart disease and cancer.

Fats—Take Care!

We've mentioned that nuts are rich in fat. The fat that we eat in our diet is perhaps one of the most important health determining factors. In recent times there has been a swing over to using a lot of the polyunsaturated seed oils such as sunflower oil, safflower oil, and soya bean oil for frying and general cooking. These oils are all very prone to oxidation, particularly when heated, and a number of researchers now have concerns that having too much of these types of oils in our diet may increase the risk of cancer. In the oxidized forms, these oils may even increase heart disease. There seems no doubt that the best oil for cooking is olive oil. Olive oil is a monounsaturated fat which means it is essentially very similar to the natural fat that our body produces. It is also one of the oils most stable during the heating process. If we are using oil on a salad or on bread (olive oil on bread is an excellent substitute for butter) it is ideal to use extra-virgin olive oil. This is the cold-pressed olive oil which is very rich in polyphenolic antioxidants, the health benefits of which we have already talked about. Extra virgin olive oil is believed to help protect against breast can-

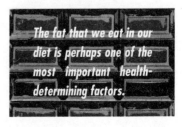

The fat that we eat in our diet is perhaps one of the most important health-determining factors.

cer. The Mediterranean countries that have a high consumption of olive oil have the lowest rates of breast cancer.

Meat?—In Moderation

So far we have not said much about meat. If using red meat, we believe it is best not to eat more than 80 g (3 oz) per day. Use only small amounts and low temperature methods of cooking such as steaming, boiling, poaching, stewing, or braising. These methods reduce the amount of oil needed to cook the meat. As you can see, we believe a chocolate lover's diet should be largely vegetarian and there are good reasons for this. John quotes

biochemist Professor Paul Walter, who recently reviewed the studies that have been done on vegetarian diets and aging. In his report, which was published in *Nutrition Reviews* in January 1997, he concluded that vegetarian diets have a much lower risk for many diseases such as obesity, car-

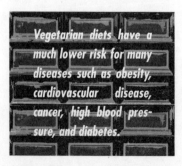

Vegetarian diets have a much lower risk for many diseases such as obesity, cardiovascular disease, cancer, high blood pressure, and diabetes.

diovascular disease, cancer, high blood pressure, and diabetes. In fact, one study of 150 young vegetarians and 150 nonvegetarians found that twice as many of the nonvegetarians had been hospitalized during the past five years and twice as many nonvegetarians as vegetarians were taking prescription medicine.

The Most Healthy Diet— The Mediterranean Diet

People living in areas of Greece and Southern Spain are noted for their longevity, and live on what is known as the Mediterranean diet, which is rich in foods that we have mentioned above; that is, whole-grain breads and pastas, lots of vegetables and legumes, fruits and nuts. They eat very few dairy products, such as butter and milk, and they eat very little red meat. They do eat moderate amounts of fish and some chicken, however.

Researchers are now finding that fish is possibly the best of all the animal foods in terms of health. In particular, the proteins in fish are believed to help lower blood pressure, and the fats in fish (the fish oils) provide essential omega 3 fatty acids. These help to protect against diabetes, heart disease, and cancer. For heart health, experts are recommending that we have about three fish meals per week.

Yogurt

Another important component of the Mediterranean diet is yogurt (the Greek type yogurt). Yogurt can be a source of what is known as "probiotic bacteria." Without certain types of bacteria, human life would not be possible. It is now known that "good" bacteria play a very important role in our health; producing vitamins, making certain nutrients such as isoflavones more available to the body, and even protecting us against harmful bacteria such as salmonella and listeria. Certain varieties are even believed to help protect against different forms of cancer (particularly cancer in the bowel) and some help lower cholesterol levels.

Eat Well, Drink Wisely, and Be Happy!

Sugar and highly refined sweets are only a very small part of the Mediterranean diet, and in our view one or two pieces of chocolate after a meal would not compromise the benefits this type of diet offers. However, part of the tradition of the Mediterranean meal time is to have a glass of wine. Red wine can be a particularly rich source of polyphenolic antioxidants which are also found in red grape juice (but without the harmful effects of alcohol). Scientists at the Harvard School of Public Health have recently pointed out that even a modest amount of alcohol may be associated with a small increase in the risk of breast cancer. So, if you're having a glass of wine, remember there are nonalcoholic wines now widely available. Have your wine in the early part of the meal and still finish off with a piece of chocolate.

Wine and chocolate are both foods that can help us feel happy. Being happy and having a positive outlook on life is a very important factor in health. In fact, a study of more than 1,000 centenarians from several countries, which was reported at the 1997 congress of the International Association of Gerontology, identified an optimistic outlook on life as the common characteristic across the group.

. . . And Don't Forget to Exercise

Another important aspect of our lifestyle is exercise. Regular exercise every day not only helps reduce the amount of fat our body will store and strengthens our heart muscle, but also helps us feel better generally. Regular exercise can

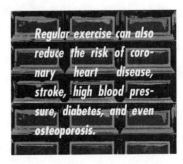

Regular exercise can also reduce the risk of coronary heart disease, stroke, high blood pressure, diabetes, and even osteoporosis.

also reduce the risk of coronary heart disease, stroke, high blood pressure, diabetes, and even osteoporosis (the weakening of the bones with age). There is also evidence that regular exercise improves our immune system and may even help the body fight some cancers. Health experts now recommend that every day we should spend at least one hour on our feet moving around, climbing stairs, walking, working in the garden, playing, or just generally keeping active. It does not need to be continuous, but throughout the day we should try to accumulate at least 60 minutes of these sorts of activities. In addition to this, we should plan some regular recreational activities for at least three times a week for at least 30 minutes or longer. These activities should be continuous and done at an intensity that brings a sweat, raises our heart rate, and has us breathing more deeply. They would include such things as brisk walking or jogging, swimming, cycling, aerobics or court sports. If we can fit it into our program, walking half an hour a day is perhaps the most natural, best all-around activity for keeping our body healthy.

. . . Or Neglect Your Spirit

Swedish botanist Linnaeus, himself a regular chocolate consumer, named the genus of the cocoa tree *theobroma*, meaning "beverage of the gods." We like to think of the cocoa tree as a gift from our Creator, a really special food. Remembering our Creator each week can also be a part of a healthy lifestyle. In recent times, the healing power of a religious faith has become increasingly recognized by scientific researchers. In 1999 Dr. Harold Koenig, Director of Duke University's Center for the Study of Religion, Spirituality, and Health, published a number of recent findings in an interesting book titled *The Healing Power of Faith—Science Explores Medicine's Last Great Frontier*. For example, Dr. David Larson, president of the U.S. National Institute for Health Care Research, and coworkers at Duke University found that people who attended religious services at least once a week, and who prayed or studied the Bible at least daily, had a consistently lower blood pressure than those who did so less frequently or not at all. They also found that the more religious patients were, the more quickly they recovered from depression. In a study of 1,718 older adults in North Carolina, the researchers found that those who attended church at least once a week had a significantly healthier immune system and improved control over stress. The Duke University scientists also found that patients aged 60 years and older who attended church weekly or more often were significantly less likely in the previous year to have been admitted to the hospital, had fewer acute hospital admissions and spent fewer days in a hospital, than those attending church less often.

This reminds me of a time when I overheard the conversation of some well-dressed schoolgirls on a train. The uniforms they were wearing told me that they attended a prestigious private girls' school in the city. Excitedly they talked about going to the Cathedral for the weekly school worship service on Thursday mornings. As I listened further, it turned out that it was a tradition to serve the students chocolate éclairs and sweet cream buns as a morning tea after the service. A case of feeding the body as well as the soul.

We believe making happy memories is one of the most important aspects of living, and the chocolate lover's lifestyle is one in which whatever you do—eating or exercising, working or worshiping—your life is enhanced by the happy inclusion of chocolate.

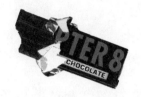

That Romantic Evening

A Fairy-tale Romance . . . Almost

Kim was just stepping out of the deliciously perfumed bath she had been luxuriating in, when she was rudely interrupted by the harsh sound of a phone ringing.

"Bother," she thought as she raced into the bedroom and picked up the receiver.

"Hi Kim, it's Rob here. I hope I wasn't interrupting anything. I just thought I'd give you a call."

Kim's heart rate increased with every word Rob spoke. Rob was the new guy at work and he was very attractive, as well as nice, and he had a good sense of humor. Kim had agonized for days about whether or not to give Rob her phone number, and he hadn't called her until now.

"Um, no, you're not interrupting anything. I was just relaxing after work," she said, stumbling over her words.

"Do you have any plans for tonight?" Rob asked.

Kim's heart rate increased further to the point where she thought she might faint, but she managed to mutter: "No, um, not tonight."

"What about dinner, then. Say around eight o'clock?"

"That would be lovely," Kim managed to say in a more sedate voice.

"Good, then. I'll pick you up at eight," said Rob.

Kim listened until she heard the phone click followed by the dial tone. Even then, she couldn't believe that Rob was asking her out for dinner, tonight!

"Oh my! What should I wear?" was the first thought racing through her distracted mind as she hurried to the closet.

While Kim was wondering what to wear, Rob was just as nervous trying to decide which flowers would be Kim's favorite. He might be the new guy, but his eyes were keen and he had noticed Kim from his first day at work. He looked at dozens of bunches before finally deciding on the traditional red roses.

At eight o'clock Rob arrived at Kim's apartment and nervously walked up to the door. He hesitated for a moment, then gave a resounding knock.

Meanwhile, Kim had been frantically searching for her favorite perfume. She'd been dreaming about tonight and how wonderful it would be. Rob would turn up at eight precisely, and offer her a ladylike-size box of chocolates. The rest of the evening would flow perfectly from there.

When she heard the knock at the door, Kim breathed deeply and checked herself one last time in the full-length mirror. Satisfied, she walked through the living room and tried to open the door calmly. Rob was standing there looking exactly as she'd imagined. She just knew that he had a box of chocolates behind his back, ready to give to her. Rob smiled at Kim and shyly held out the bunch of roses to her. Kim, however, stared at them for a minute before saying, "They're nice, Rob, really nice, but where's the box of chocolates?"

Chocolate — Why Is It So Special?

What is it about chocolate that makes us go so starry eyed and blissful, forgetting everything else around us? It's hard to believe that a food that gives women so much joy was once restricted to men. The Aztec warriors believed that cocoa gave them special energy and they used this against their enemies in battle. Cocoa drinks were also popular at weddings, and were commonly used as a nuptial aid. We are catching on to this idea in modern times. It is now quite acceptable for the happy couple to choose a double chocolate fudge mudcake for their wedding day! Men can spend just as much time choosing a bunch of flowers for us as they do choosing a box of chocolates; but we're often disappointed when we don't receive a gift of little, sweet, bite-sized pieces of heaven. Flowers *and* chocolates are very nice, too!—they are the traditional dating gifts in Western society. They make us feel special because someone has gone out of their way to help us feel happy. Even the names and shapes of chocolates can invoke feelings of happiness. Chocolate kisses not only look and taste nice, but the very thought of a kiss brings "warm, fuzzy" feelings! Not to mention the cute little heart-shaped chocolates that are so popular around Valentine's Day!

In a world where autonomy and the rights of the individual are given first preference, it's nice to see people caring about each other in this special way. It would be a shame if the one day of the year when we give special attention to our partner, Valentine's Day, never existed. I'm sure the card manufacturers wouldn't be the only ones to miss the benefits this day brings. Feeling special and wanted is a vital part of being human. It's natural to crave affection, and to want to give it. Giving someone a gift of chocolates is a way of showing them how much they mean to you. Romance is the art of making someone feel special. It's the glue that keeps two people together—that special bond of togetherness, which excludes all others. Having a healthy, happy relationship brings joy to the couple as well as those around them. It also has health benefits. People who enjoy a long-lasting, happy relationship have less stress in their lives and more energy to give life a go.

The Gender Gap—
Chocolate Divides the Sexes!

The relationship shared between chocolate and women, however, doesn't seem to be the same as between chocolate and men. Ask a group of women what a romantic evening is, and most of them will include chocolate somewhere in their description. Some will say that it is *essential* to life, and others will even go as far as to say that chocolate is better than men, or at least better than sex! Ask men the same question, and you'll probably get answers like, "She'll wear something nice," or "She'll want to be affectionate."

My husband usually answers this question with a delicate bunch of red roses and baby's breath (my favorite!), and a box of my favorite chocolates. If he's feeling exceptionally romantic, he'll take me out to dinner as well. He doesn't mind that when we go out, I usually choose the most chocolate saturated dessert on the menu.

All the restaurants that we've dined at have at least one dessert so full of chocolate that I cannot resist it. My husband usually looks at me with a quizzical expression when I squeal with delight as the Triple Chocolate Fudge Mudcake (with extra chocolate sauce and cream!) arrives at our table. I lift the fork to my mouth and take the first bite;

my eyes closing in ecstasy as I relish the moment and savor the flavor of that first sublime mouthful.

"Mmm, yum! This is fantastic!" is my first comment when I eventually float back down from chocolate heaven. Nathan just looks up from his sticky date pudding and says he's glad I like it. Like it? Like is too small a word for what I'm experiencing. So, shiny eyed, I offer him some. He hesitantly pulls my dish over to his side of the table and takes a bite. Nothing. No closed eyes, no small moans of ecstatic delight. He looks almost disappointed that this brown mound of chocolatey dessert hasn't worked the same magical effect on him that it has on me. He says he likes the cream, then goes back to his sticky date pudding. Only slightly disappointed, I retrieve my precious dessert and take another bite.

Some people might say that chocolate is God's way of reminding men of how inadequate they are! I don't think that they're inadequate exactly, but when it comes to chocolate, men just don't seem to have the appreciation for it that women do. They can, however, appreciate the happiness that this delightful food brings to their partners. The ability to appreciate someone else's happiness, even if we can't appreciate it in the same way ourselves, is one of the greatest acts of selflessness. Putting someone else's needs for pleasure on par with our own can take effort, but it is this effort that endears us to the other person. Chocolate is one way of saying to someone: "You're special. I want you to enjoy life, and be happy." Chocolate is also a sharing experience. When two people share the same experiences, it creates a bond between them. Memories shared can heighten a sense of togetherness and help to keep a couple together through times of stress. Sharing moments of tenderness over a candlelit dinner, or enjoying a secluded picnic, are just some of the pleasurable experiences couples can share together. A tender moment spent over a box of chocolates on Valentine's Day, or on an anniversary, can enhance the romance of the mood and give added delight to the occasion.

The health benefits of chocolate have been outlined in this book. When we combine a happy, fulfilling relationship with the health benefits of chocolate, we'll find that there is one more way to enjoy life to its fullest. That is what enjoying chocolate is all about! Living a healthy, balanced life, as well as caring for ourselves and others, is the main philosophy behind the chocolate lifestyle. Now you can truly believe that chocolate

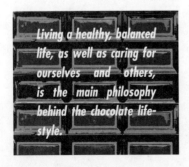

Living a healthy, balanced life, as well as caring for ourselves and others, is the main philosophy behind the chocolate lifestyle.

is good for you, and you know the reasons why living a chocolate lifestyle works. So please, don't be afraid of enjoying life to its fullest—enhance your day now, and partake in one of life's simplest but most exquisite pleasures: *chocolate!*

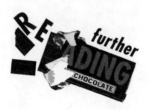

ABOUT CHOCOLATE

M. Presilla, *The New Taste of Chocolate: A Cultural and Natural History of Cacao with Recipes*, Ten Speed Press, 2001.

I. Knight (Editor), *Chocolate and Cocoa: Health and Nutrition*, Blackwell Science Ltd, Oxford, 1999.

Web Sites: www.chocolateinfo.com
            www.cocoapro.com
            www.icco.org
            www.acri-cocoa.org

ABOUT FOOD AND NUTRITION

J. Braun and B. Hornick (Editors), *The American Dietetic Association's Complete Food and Nutrition Guide*, Chronimed Publishing, Minneapolis, 1996.

J. Carper, *Food: Your Miracle Medicine: How Food Can Prevent and Cure Over 100 Symptoms and Problems*, Harper Mass Market Paperbacks, New York, 1998.

G. Kirschmann and J. Kirschmann, *Nutrition Almanac*, McGraw-Hill, New York, 1996.

ABOUT FOOD PROCESSING
J. Ashton and R. Laura, *The Perils of Progress: The Health and Environment Hazards of Modern Technology and What You Can Do About Them*, Zed Books, London, 1999.

ABOUT DIETARY FATS
A. Simopoulos and J. Robinson, *The Omega Diet: The Lifesaving Nutrition Program Based on the Diet of the Island of Crete*, HarperCollins, New York, 1999.

ABOUT DIETARY SUGARS
T. Wolever, J. Brand Brand-Miller, K. Foster-Powell, and S. Colagiuri, *The Glucose Revolution: The Authoritative Guide to the Glycemic Index—The Groundbreaking Medical Discovery*, Marlowe & Co., 1999.

ABOUT LIFESTYLE

H. Koenig, *Healing Power of Faith: How Belief and Prayer Can Help You Triumph Over Disease*, Touchstone Books, New York 2001.

K. Linamen, *Just Hand Over the Chocolate and No One Will Get Hurt*, Baker Book House, Grand Rapids, 1999.

ABOUT ROMANCE

Your favorite!

Happy Reading!